OXFORD MEDICAL PUBLICATIONS

Management of Brain-injured Children

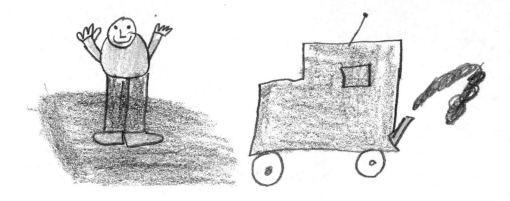

I got run over on 13th May and
I was in a coma for days and
I was in Alder Hey Hospital

John-Paul (aged 8)

Management of Brain-injured Children

Edited by

RICHARD E. APPLETON

Consultant Paediatric Neurologist

and

TONY BALDWIN

Principal Educational Psychologist
Alder Hey Children's Hospital, Liverpool, UK

Oxford New York Tokyo
OXFORD UNIVERSITY PRESS
1998

Oxford University Press, Great Clarendon Street, Oxford OX2 6DP

Oxford New York
Athens Auckland Bangkok Bogata Bombay
Buenos Aires Calcutta Cape Town Dar es Salaam
Delhi Florence Hong Kong Istanbul Karachi
Kuala Lumpur Madras Madrid Melbourne
Mexico City Nairobi Paris Singapore
Taipei Tokyo Toronto Warsaw
and associated companies in
Berlin Ibadan

Oxford is a trade mark of Oxford University Press

Published in the United States
by Oxford University Press, Inc., New York

© Oxford University Press, 1998

A catalogue record for this book is available from the British Library

Library of Congress Cataloging in Publication Data
(Data available)

ISBN 0 19 262794 5 (h/b)
ISBN 0 19 262793 7 (p/b)

Typeset by Hewer Text Composition Services, Edinburgh

Printed in Great Britain by
Biddles Ltd, Guildford & King's Lynn

Contents

Contributors

Richard E. Appleton
Consultant Paediatric Neurologist
Roald Dahl EEG Unit
ROYAL LIVERPOOL CHILDREN'S NHS TRUST (Alder Hey)
Eaton Road
LIVERPOOL
L12 2AP

Tony Baldwin
Consultant Psychologist (Educational neuropsychology)
Child Development Centre
ROYAL LIVERPOOL CHILDREN'S NHS TRUST (Alder Hey)

Colin Demellweek
Lecturer in Clinical Psychology
University Child Mental Health
ROYAL LIVERPOOL CHILDREN'S NHS TRUST (Alder Hey)

Sue Fishwick
Senior Occupational Therapist
Child Development Centre
ROYAL LIVERPOOL CHILDREN'S NHS TRUST (Alder Hey)

Jackie Gregg
Consultant Community Paediatrician
Department of Community Child Health
ROYAL LIVERPOOL CHILDREN'S NHS TRUST (Alder Hey)

Bronwen Hughes
Senior Occupational Therapist
Child Development Centre
ROYAL LIVERPOOL CHILDREN'S NHS TRUST (Alder Hey)

Eileen Kinley
Superintendent Physiotherapist
Child Development Centre
ROYAL LIVERPOOL CHILDREN'S NHS TRUST (Alder Hey)

Siobhan McMahon
Specialist Speech and Language Therapist
Department of Speech and Language Therapy
NORTH MERSEY COMMUNITY NHS TRUST

Julie Nash
Ward Manager
Neurology Ward
ROYAL LIVERPOOL CHILDREN'S NHS TRUST (Alder Hey)

Audrey O'Leary
Social Worker
c/o Roald Dahl EEG Unit
ROYAL LIVERPOOL CHILDREN'S NHS TRUST (Alder Hey)

Jane Ratcliffe
Consultant in Paediatric Intensive Care
Intensive Care Unit
ROYAL LIVERPOOL CHILDREN'S NHS TRUST (Alder Hey)

Bridget Rowland
Staff Nurse
Neurology Ward
ROYAL LIVERPOOL CHILDREN'S NHS TRUST (Alder Hey)

Jane Saltmarsh
Staff Nurse
Neurology Ward
ROYAL LIVERPOOL CHILDREN'S NHS TRUST (Alder Hey)

Heather Seddon
Head injury liaison school teacher
Hospital School
ROYAL LIVERPOOL CHILDREN'S NHS TRUST (Alder Hey)

Julie Sellars
Hospital Play Specialist
Neurology Ward
ROYAL LIVERPOOL CHILDREN'S NHS TRUST (Alder Hey)

Juliet Weston
Senior Physiotherapist
Department of Physiotherapy
ROYAL LIVERPOOL CHILDREN'S NHS TRUST (Alder Hey)

Introduction

Acquired brain injury in children is common and may follow both traumatic and non- or atraumatic insults. Although head injury is the leading cause of an acquired brain injury, non-traumatic injuries are also common. Importantly, the survival rate of children who have suffered both types of injury is increasing, in part reflecting the improved acute and resuscitative medical and surgical treatment given at the time of (and immediately following), the injury.

With this increasing survival rate there is a corresponding increase in the morbidity rate, in which children are left with significant difficulties. These difficulties can obviously range from mild to severe and transient to permanent; children may have difficulties which are limited to just one area, or more frequently, the problems are multiple and complex and have implications for physical and academic achievement and social interaction.

The primary aim in treating children who have suffered a brain injury is to rehabilitate them – literally to 'make able or competent again', and try and maximize their potential – physically, educationally and emotionally. It is clear that this process of rehabilitation must be multidisciplinary, whereby specific problems are addressed by specialists with the necessary skills. However, a multidisciplinary team is not enough; each specialist should not work in isolation but within a team to ensure an integrated, co-ordinated, and flexible approach to the rehabilitation process and to ensure that the child (and his family) are treated holistically. The team must address the changing needs of the child throughout the period of rehabilitation, and this can only be achieved if the individual team members can communicate and work effectively as a unit. It is not only the lack of specific individual skills but the absence of this co-ordinated approach, or an identified team, that impairs or even prevents adequate rehabilitation in most hospitals and community health services.

The Alder Hey head injury rehabilitation team (known as the 'HIRT') was established less than ten years ago, primarily to undertake the rehabilitation of children living in and around Liverpool who had experienced head injuries; the HIRT now receives referrals from throughout Great Britain. The team also extended its remit to include children who had suffered non-traumatic brain injuries (e.g. following a prolonged cardiac arrest, near-drowning accident or following meningitis or encephalitis); this is because the problems and needs of these children and methods of rehabilitation are often very similar to those with head injuries.

The HIRT felt that there was a need for a book which could provide a comprehensive, but practical and accessible overview and guide for any 'specialist' who is either regularly or, perhaps more importantly, only occasionally required to treat children with acquired brain injury; these 'specialists' may work within health care, education, social services or even parent support groups. The book has been written by the team members in a style and format which essentially reflects its day-to-day work pattern and which also emphasizes the multidisciplinary and integrated approach to understanding the difficulties of the brain-injured child and his family.

The book may demonstrate certain gaps and deficiences which highlight not only our, but possibly everyone's, limitations in the knowledge and understanding of acquired brain injury. *Management of Brain-Injured Children* should be regarded as a complement to the currently available specialist books which address specific problems and issues in more depth, and it is our hope and belief that it will serve as a useful and stimulating introduction to what is still a relatively under-recognized and under-resourced public (hospital and community) health problem.

ACKNOWLEDGEMENT

As one would expect, the successful completion of this book has depended on a large number of talented contibutors: most importantly the children and their families, particularly Lizzie, Paula and Charlie Pearson and John-Paul Anderson; our colleague Lewis Rosenbloom who saw the initial vision of the team; the individual authors who so eagerly and assiduously gave of their free time; Linda Finnegan for her unfailing enthusiasm and skill in typing the manuscript; and REA's wife, Jeanette and children, Sarah, James and Anna for their advice, patience and support.

R.E.A.
T.B.

Liverpool
March 1998

1

Epidemiology – incidence, causes, and severity

Richard Appleton

This chapter will briefly discuss how common brain injury, and in particular, head injury is in children, the causes of brain injuries, and how both the severity and outcome of brain injuries can be assessed and measured.

TRAUMATIC BRAIN INJURY (HEAD INJURY)

The incidence of head injury

Head injury is the most common cause of death in childhood and is a major source of handicap and disability. In 1992, reported deaths from head injuries (including skull fractures) to the Office of Population Censuses and Surveys (OPCS) totalled over 3500; 278 of these occurred in children under the age of 15 and 553 under the age of 20 years. It is important to realize that this almost certainly represents an underestimate. Furthermore, it is also obvious that this figure represents only a small fraction of all children experiencing head injury, as fortunately the majority of these children survive, although a significant number are left with residual physical and neurological problems. Nationwide, it is estimated that between 50 and 60 out of every 1000 children (i.e. between 5–6%) under the age of 14 years are admitted to hospital with a closed head injury each year. At the Royal Liverpool Children's NHS Trust, Alder Hey, our own experience revealed that, in 1995, 5081 children under 15 years of age attended the Accident and Emergency (A & E) department with a diagnosis of a head injury (including all degrees of severity); this represents approximately 2.5% of the local childhood population which is served by our hospital. Of these 5081 children 400 (almost 8%) required admission to hospital for a minimum of 24 hours. These figures are similar to those reported elsewhere within Great Britain and also in the United States.

The causes of head injury

The majority of head injuries to children occur as a result of the following (Kraus *et al.* 1986, 1990, Sharples *et al.* 1990*b*; Ward 1995):

- road traffic accidents where the child is either a pedestrian (most common), a passenger in a car, or a cyclist (least common)
- falls from buildings/play equipment/trees
- injuries from objects (e.g. golf club/ball, bricks/stones, firearm [air- or shotgun])
- non-accidental injury (child abuse)
- sports-related injury (e.g. horse-riding, rugby, cycling, skate-boarding or roller-blading, rock climbing)
- epileptic fits and other causes of loss of consciousness

Age

In the first year of life, non-accidental injury (child abuse) is almost certainly the most common cause of both moderate and severe traumatic brain injury. In middle childhood (between the ages of 5 and 12 years), the most common causes would include road traffic accidents where the child is usually a pedestrian or cyclist (often involved with playing on or near busy roads), and taking part in dangerous activities including climbing trees or roofs of buildings and games of 'chicken' or 'dare' (this involves children 'daring' each other to run across busy roads at the last minute before oncoming vehicles). From 12 years upwards, more common causes include road traffic accidents involving cyclists and sports/games (Kraus *et al.* 1990; Lundar and Nestvold 1985; Rivara 1984, 1994, Ward 1995). The use of alcohol (and its increasing consumption) contributes to a number of teenager-related head injuries – whatever the cause.

It is not surprising that at least half of all head injuries in children will occur during the course of play, much of it unsupervised (Craft *et al.* 1972; Sharples *et al.* 1990*b*). This has implications for the possible prevention of head injuries.

Sex

As with all types and causes of head trauma, males have approximately twice the rate of brain injuries than females (Fig. 1.1). These differences appear early, even in the preschool years (including child abuse or non-accidental injury), and almost certainly reflect a difference in behaviour (and maturity) between boys and girls as well as differences in exposure to specific hazards which result in head injury - i.e. boys take part in more dangerous activities (Rivara 1994).

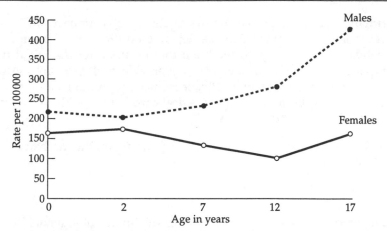

Fig. 1.1 Age-specific brain injury rates per 100 000 by gender, San Diego County, California, USA, 1981. (Reproduced with permission from Rivara, F. P. (1994). *Pediatric Annals*, **23**, 12–17).

Socio-economic status

Evidence from both this country (Sharples 1990*b*) and other countries including the United States (Kraus *et al.* 1990; Rivara 1990), perhaps not surprisingly, has shown that children from poorer backgrounds (reflecting a lower socio-economic status of their parents) have both an increased inci-dence of, and mortality from, head injury. There will clearly be many reasons for this, including reduced supervision, increased exposure to hazardous situations (particularly in traffic-intense and relatively derelict inner-city areas) and a reduced knowledge and understanding of preventative and avoidance strategies.

Additional factors which may also contribute to the risk and cause of head injuries in this population are pre-existing learning difficulties or behaviour problems, or both, which may predispose these children to experiencing injuries. This has been our experience, with almost three-quarters of over 110 children with head injuries having evidence of pre-injury cognitive or behavioural dysfunction; this has been described previously (Bijur *et al.* 1990; Ward 1995).

It is also likely that there will be ethnic differences between different racial groups; this may not necessarily be a primary effect but secondary to other variables, including socio-economic status.

Pathogenesis of brain injury following traumatic head injury

It is important to realize that brain injury, and therefore brain damage may arise by two mechanisms which may occur singly or in combination:

(1) primary - i.e. damage that occurs at the time of impact and which is irreversible. The type of damage depends on the type of trauma

(2) secondary - ie: damage to the brain that occurs after the initial trauma (impact) and which *may* be both preventable and reversible. Any secondary damage can, theoretically, be reduced or minimized by rapid and optimal resuscitation and acute medical care following the initial trauma (Sharples *et al.* 1990*a*).

Both of these can be further classified, depending on the mechanism of the injury/damage.

Primary

These include skull fractures, lacerations of the brain, subarachnoid haemorrhage, haematomas (subdural, epidural, and extradural,) and cerebral contusion.

An alternative way of classifying the primary injury is by dividing it into either penetrating (such as occurs when the child is struck by, or falls on, an object) or non-penetrating (which occurs when an acceleration–deceleration force causes shearing stresses between different layers of brain). Non-penetrating injuries are the more common type of mechanism of injury in children and often occur without any accompanying skull fracture or external sign of injury to the head. The shearing stresses may cause severe damage to a large number of nerve cells (axons and neurons), and may also tear or rupture blood vessels, the olfactory nerve (resulting in anosmia or the loss of the sense of smell), and the pituitary stalk (resulting in transient or permanent hormonal deficiencies, particularly diabetes insipidus). Not surprisingly, severe acceleration–deceleration injuries with irreversible damage to the neurons and axons (called diffuse axonal injury), may result in very severe neurological deficits. Even milder acceleration–deceleration injuries may cause a temporary neurological deficit, which is often referred to as concussion. There is increasing evidence that even after these so-called 'mild' injuries, subtle neurological and psychological effects (primarily on concentration and attention span and behaviour) can occur and may persist for months or even years. In these 'milder' head injuries imaging of the brain with magnetic resonance imaging (MRI) may show evidence of diffuse axonal injury which is not visible using computerised tomography (CT) (Mittl *et al.* 1994).

Secondary

There are a number of different causes of secondary brain damage, including:

• intracranial haematoma (subdural, extradural, or epidural)

- cerebral oedema (brain swelling)
- cerebral ischaemia (due to increased intracranial pressure, or due to systemic hypotension resulting from haemorrhage from other traumatic organs)
- cerebral hypoxia (arising from respiratory failure due to either damage to the lungs or because of raised intracranial pressure causing compression of the brainstem where the control of breathing is located).

Intracranial haematomas occur less frequently in children than in adults; the presence of a subdural haematoma in a young child (under 2 or 3 years of age) should raise the suspicion of non-accidental injury.

Finally, the secondary effects of a brain injury cannot – and should not – be underestimated. These effects contribute significantly to both the mortality and morbidity of traumatic brain injury and emphazise the importance of rapid resuscitation and good medical care, particularly in the first hour or so (the 'golden hour') following the injury.

ATRAUMATIC OR NON-TRAUMATIC BRAIN INJURY

It is important to realize that brain damage may also, in contrast to traumatic brain injury (TBI), be caused by non-traumatic or atraumatic brain injury (ABI). These injuries may be caused by a large number of different disorders:

- as a complication of meningitis or encephalitis
- as a complication of a hypoxic–ischaemic cerebral insult (caused by a reduction in blood flow and therefore the supply of oxygen to the brain). This may occur in the following:
  - strokes
  - near-drowning accidents
  - asphyxiation/suffocation (as may occur as a complication of the inhalation of smoke in a fire)
  - during any surgical procedure, particularly cardiac (heart) surgery, and neurosurgery for the removal of brain tumours
  - in prolonged status epilepticus (when an epileptic convulsion lasts more than 60 minutes.)
- as a complication of diabetes (due to hypo- or hyperglycaemia)
- as a complication of some other metabolic or biochemical impairment.

These atraumatic brain injuries are not uncommon but there is no accurate information as to their incidence (i.e. how many children experience an ABI per year) or their prevalence (i.e. how many children admitted to hospital have an ABI at any given point in time).

Our own experience at Alder Hey suggests that when one considers all causes of atraumatic brain injury together, the incidence and prevalence of *significant* ABI may be as high, or even higher, than TBI. This pattern seems to have been emerging over the past couple of years (Fig. 1.2 and 1.3). However, it must be emphasised that these data refer only to a highly selected group of children (those actually referred to the multidisciplinary Head Injury Rehabilitation Team [called the HIRT] at Alder Hey) and not necessarily to all children admitted to Alder Hey with either a TBI or ABI. Clearly, TBI will be more common than ABI if one considers all head injuries, irrespective of severity.

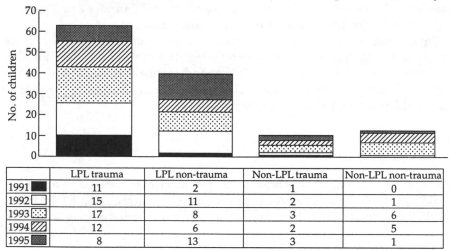

	LPL trauma	LPL non-trauma	Non-LPL trauma	Non-LPL non-trauma
1991 ■	11	2	1	0
1992 □	15	11	2	1
1993 ▨	17	8	3	6
1994 ▨	12	6	2	5
1995 ▨	8	13	3	1

Fig. 1.2   Origin and type of children treated from 1991 to 1995. LPL refers to Liverpool.

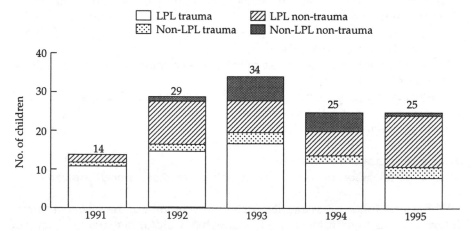

Fig. 1.3   Yearly total number of children treated from 1991 to 1995. LPL refers to Liverpool.

It has been suggested that in an average health care district within Great Britain, per year six children with a TBI and four children with an ABI will require 'rehabilitation'. Clearly, these figures are a very crude estimate and will obviously depend on the defining criteria for 'rehabilitation' and almost certainly therefore will represent an underestimate of children requiring varying degrees of rehabilitative resources and facilities.

ARE TBI AND ABI BECOMING MORE COMMON?

There is very little information on this issue, but both are almost certainly increasing in frequency. Evidence from Newcastle (although, admittedly rather old) showed a sixfold increase between 1950 and 1970 in the numbers of children admitted with TBI (Craft *et al.* 1972). A number of factors may have been responsible for this increase including:

- a *real* increase in head injuries due to:
  - a larger paediatric population
  - an increased number and use of motor vehicles and cycles
  - a reduction in supervision of children by parents
  - changes in social attitudes (whether at home or at school)
- an *apparent* increase in head injuries, due to:
  - a reduction in criteria requiring or necessitating admission to hospital
  - an increased rate of reporting of children with head injuries.

One important additional factor, which will almost certainly be contributing to an increasing number of children surviving severe head injuries, is an improvement in resuscitation and acute management at the time of the injury; previously, many of these children would have died, but an increasing number are surviving (but with severe neurological and other medical complications) as a result of improved roadside treatment and intensive care facilities (Sharples *et al.* 1990*a*).

The number of children with ABI is almost certainly increasing for the same reason – namely, due to the improved management of acute encephalopathies (including meningitis and encephalitis) and improved anaesthesia and intraoperative monitoring during surgical procedures.

THE SEVERITY OF BRAIN INJURIES (TBI AND ABI)

Although there are relatively good data on the overall incidence and prevalence of head injuries in children, there is less reliable information on the different grades of severity of head injury. This may be due to a number of factors, including the variable reporting of the severity of the head injury (i.e. the information is not available) and inconsistency in the method of measuring the severity of the head injury. This applies particularly to 'minor' head injuries. These 'minor' head injuries are obviously far more common than 'major' injuries and may be initially considered as relatively unimportant (or even ignored), but nevertheless may be followed by significant cognitive and behavioural sequelae (Casey *et al.* 1986, Wrightson *et al.* 1995). Currently, there are many ways of assessing the severity of a traumatic brain injury:

- the Glasgow Coma Scale (Box 1.1) (Jennett and Teasdale 1981)
- the Glasgow Coma Scale for children (Box 1.2) (Simpson *et al.* 1991)
- the Abbreviated Injury Scale (Box 1.3)

(these two are probably the most commonly used measures, primarily because of their ease of use and also because they are standardized)

- other (often locally or regionally and not nationally) - devised coma scales
- the duration of any coma (Box 1.4)
- the duration of any post-traumatic amnesia or 'PTA' (PTA is defined as a period of variable length after closed head trauma during which the patient is confused, disorientated, describes retrograde amnesia, and is unable to remember and recall new information)
- duration of ventilatory support.

Box 1.1 Glasgow Coma Scale*

		Score
Eyes open (E)	Spontaneously	4
	To speech	3
	To pain	2
	Do not open	1
Best verbal response (V)	Orientated	5
	Confused	4
	Inappropriate words	3
	Incomprehensible sounds	2
	None	1
Best motor response (M)	Obeys commands	6
	Localizes pain	5
	Withdraws to pain	4
	Flexes limbs to pain	3
	Extends limbs to pain	2
	None	1
	Total	15

*Coma score = E + V + M

Box 1.2 Paediatric Glasgow Coma Scale

	> 1 year	< 1 year	Score
Eyes open	Spontaneously	Spontaneously	4
	To command	To shout	3
	To pain	To pain	2
	No response	No response	1
Best verbal response	Orientated and converses	Appropriate words/phrases	5
	Disorientated and converses	Inappropriate words	4
	Inappropriate words	Cries	3
	Incomprehensible sounds	Grunts	2
	No response	No response	1
Best motor response	Obeys commands	–	5
	Localises pain	Localises oain	4
	Flexion to pain	Flexion to pain	3
	Extension to pain	Extension to pain	2
	No response	No response	1

Normal aggregate scores < 6 months 12
6–12 months 12
1–2 years 13
2–5 years 14
> 5 years 14

Box 1.3 Abbreviated Injury Scale

Code number	Severity	Brain Injury Example
1	Minor	Concussion but awake on initial observation
2	Moderate	Concussion with minimum loss of consciousness
3	Serious	Cerebral contusion
4	Severe	Subdural haematoma
5	Critical	Diffuse brain injury
6	Unsurvivable	Laceration of brain stem
7	Unknown	

Box 1.4 Duration of coma and severity of the head injury
- less than 20 minutes – 'mild'
- 20 minutes to 6 hours – 'moderate'
- 6 hours to 48 hours – 'severe'
- over 48 hours – 'very severe'

Measures of severity are important as there are relatively good correlations between the degree of head injury and neurological outcome in terms of disability. The Glasgow Coma Scale and period of post-traumatic amnesia (PTA) are, arguably, the easiest and most frequently used for correlating severity with outcome. There is also a corresponding Glasgow Outcome Scale which is used to measure the outcome of brain injury and this can be applied to both children and adults. The outcome levels are:

- good recovery
- moderate disability
- severe disability
- persistent vegetative state
- death.

(Clearly, the first three of these outcome levels are rather subjective and should only be regarded as a crude assessment of outcome.)

Unfortunately, the use (and therefore value) of the period of PTA to predict outcome is very limited in young children because memory may be difficult, if not impossible, to assess.

As yet, there is no separate measure (similar to the Glasgow Coma Scale) for children (or for adults) who have suffered an ABI. This is largely due to the fact that the causes of ABI are multiple and heterogeneous and it is therefore difficult to score them using a single scale. However, the scales used for trauma are still be of value in assessing the severity of atraumatic coma.

REFERENCES

Bijur, P. E., Haslum, M., and Golding, J. (1990). Cognitive and behavioural sequelae of mild head injury in children. *Pediatrics*, 86, 337–44.

Casey, R., Ludwig, S., and McCormick, M.C. (1986). Morbidity following minor head trauma in children. *Pediatrics*, 78, 497–502.

Craft, A., Shaw, D., and Cartlidge, N. (1972). Head injuries in children. *British Medical Journal*, 4, 200–3.

Jennett, B and Teasdale, G. (1981). *Management of head injuries*, pp. 258–63. F.A. Davis Co., Philadelphia, USA.

Kraus, J. F., Fife, D, Cox, P., Ramstein, K., and Conroy, C. (1986). Incidence, severity, and external causes of pediatric brain injury. *American Journal of Diseases in Children*, 140, 687–93.

Kraus, J. F., Rock, A, and Hemyari, P. (1990). Brain injuries among infants, children, adolescents and young adults. *Americal Journal of Diseases in Children*, 144, 684–91.

Lundar, T. and Nestvold, K. (1985). Pediatric head injuries caused by traffic accidents. A prospective study with 5 year follow-up. *Child's Nervous System*, 1, 24–8.

Mittl, R., Grossman, R., Hiehle, T., *et al.* (1994). Prevalence of MR evidence of diffuse axonal injury in patients with mild head injury and normal head CT findings. *American Journal of Neuroradiology*, 15, 1583–9.

Rivara, F. P. (1984). Childhood injuries. III. Epidemiology of non-motor vehicle head trauma. *Developmental Medicine and Child Neurology*, 26, 81–7.

Rivara, F. P. (1990). Child pedestrian injuries in the United States. *American Journal of Diseases in Children*, 144, 692–6.

Rivara, F. P. (1994). Epidemiology and prevention of pediatric traumatic brain injury. *Pediatric Annals*, **23**, 12-17.

Sharples, P. M., Storey, A., Aynsley-Green, A., and Eyre, J. A. (1990a). B Avoidable factors contributing to death of children with head injury. *British Medical Journal*, **300**, 87-91.

Sharples, P. M., Storey, A., Aynsley-Green, A., and Eyre, J. A. (1990b). Causes of fatal childhood accidents involving head injury in the Northern region, 1979–86. *British Medical Journal*, **301**, 1193–7.

Simpson, D. A., Cockington, R. A., Hanieh, A., Raftos, J., and Reilly, P. L. (1991). Head injuries in infants and young children: the value of the paediatric coma scale. *Childs Nervous System*, **7**, 183–90.

Ward, J. D. (1995). Pediatric issues in head trauma. *New Horizons*, **3**, 539–45.

Wrightson, P., McGinn, V., and Gronwall, D. (1995). Mild head injury in preschool children: evidence that it can be associated with a persisting cognitive defect. *Journal of Neurology, Neurosurgery and Psychiatry*, **59**, 375–80.

2

Resuscitation and acute treatment of brain injuries (traumatic and atraumatic)

Jane Ratcliffe

The aim of this chapter is to provide an overview of the principles of management and to emphasize the importance of adequate initial resuscitation and the optimization of cardiovascular parameters, to reduce the incidence of secondary brain injury.

Although there are different mechanisms of acute brain injury with very different outcomes, the initial management and goals of treatment are the same. Illustrative examples of some of the types of acute brain injury will indicate why the neurological outcome is directly related to the aetiology of the insult. Rapid resuscitation and intensive care management may significantly improve the overall outcome in certain types of acute brain injury.

RESUSCITATION

Acute brain injury is associated with focal or widespread damage to the brain. This results in impairment of the normal autoregulation of cerebral blood flow in the damaged areas of brain. The aim of treatment is to maintain adequate cerebral perfusion (circulation of blood) to uninjured areas of brain, thus protecting them from the secondary damage of hypoxia (reduced or absent oxygen) and ischaemia (reduced or absent blood supply). The resuscitation protocol follows the ABCD sequence: **airway, breathing, circulation** and **disability** assessment.

A: The airway may be obstructed by blood, vomit, or the tongue falling back. Often the latter may be alleviated by lifting the jaw forward. Facial injuries may produce swelling which could compromise the airway and are an indication for early endotracheal intubation. For traumatic injuries, the cervical spine is assumed to be damaged until proved otherwise and is protected by stabilization of the neck in the midline, a position which must be maintained during intubation.

B: Adequacy of ventilation is essential for the prevention of secondary damage to the brain. Continuous oxygen saturation monitoring, end-tidal carbon dioxide monitoring (a continuous means of measuring carbon dioxide production and excretion), and blood gas analysis should complement what has been assessed visually as adequate ventilation. Both hypoxia and carbon dioxide retention are associated with cerebral vasodilatation, which immediately increases cerebral blood volume and thus increases the volume of the intracranial contents. This has profound effects on the swollen brain and will affect cerebral perfusion pressure (CPP), which is the mean arterial blood pressure minus the intracranial pressure.

C: Vascular access should be with large cannulae so that fluids can be infused rapidly. Intraosseous infusions (infusions directly into the bone marrow cavity) are very useful in establishing vascular access in hypovolaemic (reduced circulating blood volume) children. Blood pressure may be maintained for some time despite severe hypovolaemia; cardiac output being the product of heart rate and stroke volume (volume of blood pumped at each contraction of the heart muscle). Volume loading with rapid infusions of 4.5% albumin in 10ml/kg aliquots should be carried out with pulse rate and blood pressure measurements. Capillary refill greater than 3 seconds is an indication for further volume loading in children with acute brain injuries. Despite adequate volume loading and control of haemorrhage, blood pressure may remain low and the patient may require inotropic support (drugs used to increase the force of contraction of the heart) with dobutamine, dopamine, or in intractable cases, adrenaline. The requirement for the latter may be an indication of very severe brain injury or 'spinal shock' secondary to damage to the spinal cord.

D: The assessment of disability requires a detailed clinical examination to evaluate all injuries sustained during trauma. An X-ray skeletal survey, ultrasound and computerized tomography (CT) scan of the chest and abdomen may reveal additional pathology. There is no place for undertaking a CT brain scan in a child who is only partially resuscitated and stabilized. Neurological deterioration is more likely to be the result of hypovolaemia and hypotension (low blood pressure), than the presence of an acute extradural haematoma (collection of blood in the extradural space which compresses the brain) (Fig. 2.1), in such circumstances. In non-traumatic acute brain dysfunction, clinical examination may reveal a rash indicating, for example, meningococcal septicaemia, or a stiff neck (meningism) suggesting meningitis.

The Glasgow Coma Score (GCS), or modified GCS for young children, is used as an acute and ongoing tool to monitor the level of consciousness and make decisions with regard to management. A GCS of eight or lower is widely agreed to be the level at which patients are actively managed with endotracheal intubation and controlled ventilation (artificial ventilation). Children with a GCS above this level may need to be intubated and ventilated in order to obtain accurate diagnostic information from CT brain scans.

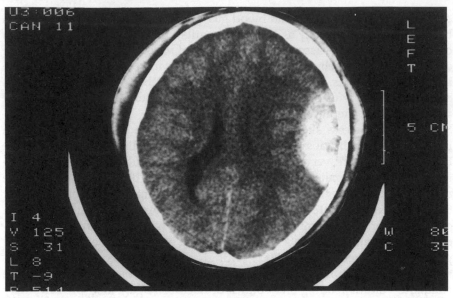

Fig 2.1 CT scan of an acute extradural haematoma with compression of the ipsilateral cerebral ventricle and midline shift.

PATHOPHYSIOLOGY OF BRAIN INJURY

Intracranial pressure

Intracranial pressure (ICP) varies with age – 0–5 mmHg up to 2 years of age; 0–10 mmHg below 5 years; and 0–5 mmHg for older children and adults (Welch 1980). It rises transiently with coughing and straining. Pathological increases in ICP occur when the volume of intracranial contents rises within the skull.

Although infants may be able to increase the cranial volume by spreading of the cranial sutures, this mechanism is restricted to more chronic or gradual increases in intracranial pressure. Intracranial mass lesions can be grouped into focal or generalized lesions or a combination of both. Blood, intracranial tumours, and obstructive hydrocephalus are examples of the former, whereas cell death secondary to hypoxia or ischaemia causes widespread cerebral oedema. Infants who have had a whiplash shaking injury (e.g. sustained during a non-accidental injury) may have features of both. The brain has limited ability to adapt to increases of intracranial volume, after which the intracranial pressure rises acutely. The brain can reduce its volume by reducing the cerebrospinal fluid (CSF) volume and the intracranial blood volume. Herniation of the cranial contents downwards into the spinal cord is the consequence of acutely raised intracranial pressure. The brainstem descends towards the foramen magnum and the compression interferes with its blood supply, causing ischaemia and obstruction to the normal flow of CSF.

Cerebral perfusion pressure and cerebral blood flow

The cerebral perfusion pressure (CPP) is defined as the difference between mean arterial pressure and ICP. Cerebral blood flow (CBF) is affected by ICP, cerebral metabolic rate, and blood oxygen and carbon dioxide tensions. The brain's energy source is oxidative phosphorylation (metabolism using oxygen) of glucose. Interference with cerebral energy provision results in rapid and irreversible neuronal cell death.

The average normal CBF has been calculated as 50 ml per 100 g of brain tissue per minute and the normal cerebral oxygen uptake rate as 3 ml per 100 g of brain tissue per minute. Cerebral blood flow is maintained at a constant level within a wide range of blood pressures by vasodilatation (dilatation of blood vessels) when blood pressure falls and progressive vasoconstriction as it rises. At lower pressures, CBF falls to zero and at higher pressures, cerebral oedema occurs. This cerebral autoregulation may be impaired in damaged areas of brain.

Cerebral blood flow in relation to arterial oxygen and carbon dioxide tensions

Low oxygen saturations cause an increase in CBF but only when the partial pressure of oxygen (pO_2) in the blood falls to 50 mmHg; at a pO_2 level of 30 mmHg, CBF increases threefold. There is relatively little decrease of CBF in response to high oxygen tensions.

CBF rises with increases of arterial partial pressure of carbon dioxide (pCO_2) and doubles when the pCO_2 increases from 40 mmHg to 80 mmHg. Cerebral vasoconstriction occurs when the arterial pCO_2 falls and CBF halves when the pCO_2 is reduced from 40 mmHg to 20 mmHg.

Changes in arterial carbon dioxide tension also affect the cerebral blood volume (CBV). Lowering pCO_2 will reduce the CBV and is a mechanism for reducing raised ICP.

INTENSIVE CARE MANAGEMENT OF THE ACUTELY BRAIN INJURED CHILD

The principles of management are the same whatever the nature of the brain injury but the outcome depends on the underlying cause. Whether or not there is a suspected neck injury, the head should be maintained in a neutral position with the body. If the patient is moved, it should be by 'log-rolling'. In terms of the head injury, supine is the optimal position, with a maximum of 30 degrees of head and upper-body elevation. The immobility related to sedation and muscle relaxants will predispose to pressure area damage and a chest infection; therefore, 'log-rolling' to 30 degrees from the horizontal plane may be useful.   Metabolic rate is increased by a raised central body temperature. Active cooling to 36°C is useful in severe head injuries. There are specialized electronic beds, some of which have the ability to cool the patient, available for paediatric patients to avoid pressure area damage.

Intracranial pressure monitoring

Knowledge of the actual intracranial pressure is essential for the management of moderately severe and severe head injuries caused by trauma, and may also be of use in some metabolic conditions associated with raised intracranial pressure. In conditions secondary to a hypoxic ischaemic encephalopathy, for example after drowning or a cardiac arrest, the degree of cerebral oedema will relate to the neuronal damage and the measurement of intracranial pressure will not influence the predictably poor outcome.

A CT scan may give the impression of raised intracranial pressure by showing compressed cerebral ventricles and loss of the normal sulcal pattern (the convolutional arrangement of cortical tissue over the surface of the brain). Direct measurement of intracranial pressure can assist in the protection of the brain from surges in intracranial pressure and can also give guidance for the timing of follow up CT scans and weaning from ventilatory support. The insertion of a fine fibre-optic catheter into the brain substance or actually into a cerebral ventricle, through a burr hole, will allow direct measurement of intracranial pressure as well as drainage of cerebrospinal fluid in the case of the latter. These fibre-optic catheters are easier to insert and have a very low incidence of complications such as bleeding. Such intracranial pressure monitoring can be linked to the bedside monitor so that a continuous measurement and waveform of cerebral perfusion pressure is obtained.

Controlled ventilation and intracranial pressure

The ability to control some acute rises in intracranial pressure by reducing pCO_2 by hyperventilation and reduction of cerebral blood flow led to the practice of managing patients being ventilated with a low pCO_2. Research has shown that such a practice may lead to inappropriate vasoconstriction for the metabolic requirements of the uninjured areas of brain and therefore a less favourable outcome (Muizelaar *et al*, 1991). Research suggests that the pCO_2 should be maintained at the lower end of the normal range, i.e. 35 mmHg. This is facilitated by using continuous end tidal CO_2 monitoring.

Rises in ICP may occur during coughing and painful stimuli; the use of muscle relaxants will minimize rises in ICP related to coughing but adequate sedation is required to reduce the effects of unpleasant external stimuli. Tachycardia associated with increased blood pressure during interventions suggests inadequate sedation.

Convulsions

There is an increased incidence of seizures following head injury. The use of anticonvulsants routinely is controversial. There is no evidence that their prophylactic use will affect the long-term outcome with regard to epilepsy. One or certainly two convulsions, which have occurred following the head injury, justify the use of an anticonvulsant to try to prevent further convulsions. One reason for using an anticonvulsant is that convulsions can cause a rise in ICP which may adversely affect CBF, contributing to further neuronal damage. Phenytoin is the drug of first choice in children; firstly, because it can be given intravenously, thereby quickly achieving adequate concentrations in the blood, and secondly, because it is non-sedative and has a shorter half life than phenobarbitone. In children in whom muscle relaxants are used, major convulsions are usually evident from changes in pupillary size, tachycardia and increases in blood pressure.

Fluid management

Normal saline is used preferentially in head injuries, except in young infants who may become hypoglycaemic without dextrose in the infusion fluid. In this group additional dextrose can be added to saline. Dextrose, when metabolized, becomes free water and may diffuse into cells within the brain and thus contribute to increased cerebral oedema. Fluid is restricted to 60 or 70% of normal maintenance requirements. Maintenance requirements are 100 ml/kg for the first 10 kg body weight, 50 ml/kg for the second 10 kg and 20 ml/kg for each subsequent 10 kg. A central venous line to measure central venous pressure (CVP) is essential for accurate fluid management. Further boluses of 4.5% albumin or blood may be required to restore the CVP to normal.

Mannitol is an osmotic diuretic used to acutely dehydrate the brain when the ICP remains severely raised or when there are clinical signs of brainstem herniation (downward movement of the cerebrum into the spinal cord). It will have an effect on normal brain tissue by causing an osmotic diuresis (withdrawal into the circulation of water from cells along an osmotic gradient) and this may interfere with the functioning of undamaged brain. Other diuretics (drugs to promote water excretion), such as frusemide may also be used as an adjunct to treatment.

Inotropic support

A low or even normal blood pressure may be inadequate to maintain the cerebral perfusion pressure in a patient with raised ICP. If the CVP is within the normal range, inotropic drugs in the form of dopamine or dobutamine may be used. In patients in whom there is damage to the spinal cord, inappropriate vasodilatation may occur with associated severe hypotension, 'spinal shock'. In these circumstances, adrenaline may be necessary.

Barbiturates

Barbiturates may be used to treat raised ICP but in turn will suppress neurological function and the electroencephalogram (EEG). They reduce both cerebral blood flow and cerebral metabolic rate. In status epilepticus, which can produce raised ICP, barbiturate-induced coma is rational. There is no benefit from using barbiturates as a treatment after global cerebral ischaemia. There are associated problems, in particular with blood pressure, and the use of barbiturates should be weighed against the potential benefits. The clinical tests to establish brainstem death cannot be carried out in the presence of barbiturates, even when measured concentrations have fallen into the 'normal' therapeutic range.

Steroids

Steroids are ineffective in acute brain injury unless there is a brain tumour with associated oedema. Their anti-inflammatory properties may increase the risk of infection and they may cause inappropriate hypertension.

Imaging in acute brain injury

Computerised tomography scanning of the brain is the technique most widely used. It is dangerous to undertake CT scanning in a patient who is not fully resuscitated and stabilized. If there is severe haemorrhage in the chest or abdomen, portable echocardiography and ultrasonography can be carried out while resuscitation continues. If it is not possible to obtain satisfactory images of a child with a potentially serious head injury because of movement or distress, intubation and ventilation may be necessary. High resolution ultrasonography of the brain in the young infant with a whiplash shaking injury may demonstrate cortical shearing damage (Jaspan *et al*, 1992).

Magnetic resonance imaging (MRI) has not been shown to have any significant advantages above CT scanning of the brain in the acute situation, but is valuable in longer- term follow-up. However, it is very useful in the assessment of spinal cord damage.

CT scanning can indicate that ICP is raised when there is reduction in size of the ventricles and basal cisterns and flattening of the cerebral sulci. However, the absence of these features does not mean that the ICP is normal. In a patient who is being managed by controlled ventilation, paralysed and sedated for presumed raised ICP, who does not have an intracranial pressure monitoring device *in situ*, a repeat CT scan after 48 hours may be useful. If there is clinical neurological deterioration, including signs of acute brainstem herniation, treatment with hyperventilation, mannitol, and frusemide should be started and an urgent CT scan obtained.

Cerebral function monitoring

Continuous single channel electroencephalogram recordings (CFAM) may give information about convulsive activity in patients who have been given muscle relaxants. Electroencephalogram (EEG) recordings may provide valuable information on both the presence of convulsions and the normality of brain electrical activity. Visual and sensory evoked responses can also be measured and give an indication of cerebral function when muscle relaxants are used.

New theories of brain resuscitation

Acute brain injury results in death of a variable number of brain cells, both neurones and neural connective tissue. There is damage to the blood–brain barrier with escape of water and plasma as a component of the oedema. Acute breakdown of cells may result in the release of cellular ions, for example calcium, which may induce vascular spasm of cerebrovascular smooth muscle and neurotransmitters. These may in turn damage other cells which are initially unaffected by the primary acute brain insult.

Attention has been focused on the time of reperfusion after a period of ischaemia. Anaerobic metabolism of glucose (metabolism of glucose without oxygen) produces lactic acid and in animal studies this has been shown to be detrimental to recovery of the ischaemic brain (Kalimo *et al*, 1981). There are physical effects related to sluggish flow of blood in small blood vessels, such as capillary sludging and platelet aggregation which may progress to permanent ischaemia and cerebral infarction.

Acute brain injury research is concentrating on the development of drugs which can improve microvascular perfusion or which can bind to, or block the effects of, potentially deleterious substances released during or immediately after brain injury – thereby reducing the damage caused by the primary injury.

ACUTE BRAIN TRAUMA

Road-traffic accidents

Child pedestrians and cyclists are likely to sustain a greater degree of head injury for a given impact velocity than adults because of the mechanism of the brain injury. The key variables are the speed of the vehicle and the weight of the child. The lighter the child, the more likely it is for the impact to fling the child into the air, resulting in a greater force of impact with the road and an acute whiplash type of injury.

The CT scan appearances reflect the mode of injury. A single impact may result in an underlying contusion. There may be a 'contre coup' effect with additional damage remote from the impact site. The more complex injury, which involves the child being flung into the air by the vehicle, may result in widespread intracerebral damage. In addition to contusion underlying the impact site, the effects of the acceleration and abrupt deceleration produce a spectrum of injuries related to the shearing forces on brain tissue. There may be diffuse intracerebral bleeding and widespread cerebral oedema resulting from brain tissue death (Fig. 2.2). The consequences of cerebral oedema may

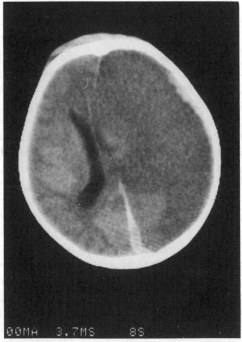

Fig 2.2 CT scan of an acute head injury with severe unilateral cerebral oedema, compression of the ipsilateral cerebral ventricle, midline shift, a small subdural haematoma and an extracranial haematoma.

be raised intracranial pressure, a fall in cerebral perfusion pressure, progressive hypoxia and ischaemia, and further brain tissue death.

The shaken-infant syndrome

This form of non-accidental injury is seen almost exclusively in children under 2 years of age and is most devastating in children under 1 year of age. Young infants have a relatively large head and a small neck with weak musculature. The nature of the injury has two components, the physical injury and secondary effects related to delay in presentation to medical attention.

The trigger for such shaking episodes is usually described as inconsolable crying. The duration of the shaking episode, where admitted, may be described as very short, e.g. less than a minute, but it is the force of the shaking which is a crucial factor in the severity of the injury produced. The infant is grasped around the upper trunk and shaken. The head flops in other directions in addition to the predominant to and fro movement. A flailing movement of the limbs occurs and characteristic appearances of bony damage may be produced in the growth plates of the wrists and ankles. At the end of the shaking episode the infant may be flung onto a hard or soft surface. Therefore there may be an associated limb or skull fracture.

The mechanism of the brain injury is acceleration of the head during the shaking episode. This causes tearing of bridging veins on the surface of the brain with the development of subdural haematomas (haemorrhages) (American Academy of Pediatrics 1993). There is diffuse intracerebral haemorrhage reflecting the severe rotational forces which are generated. It is now accepted that there does not need to be an acute deceleration at the end of a shaking episode to produce the brain lesions.

The grasping of the chest has two effects. There may be bruises where the child is grasped but often there is no mark. Rib fractures may be produced by squeezing of the chest and they may not become obvious on chest X-ray until the formation of callus (healing new bone) at about a week after the injury. The chest compression also effects venous return from the head and there is acutely raised ICP during the shaking episode. This, together with the severe rotational forces, produces retinal haemorrhages which may extend into the vitreous humour (gelatinous content of the eye globe) and along the optic nerve sheath. These retinal haemorrhages may lead to scarring and loss of visual acuity or blindness.

The second component of the shaken infant syndrome is the secondary effects produced by the shaking and the delay in seeking medical attention. The effect of shaking is to produce an alteration of conscious level. The perpetrator may believe that the infant is asleep rather than unconscious. The acute brain injury will, over a varying time course related to the severity of the injury, lead to clinical signs of cerebral irritation and swelling which may cause convulsions or cessation of breathing. The cerebral bleeding will result in acute anaemia and circulatory shock. The clinical features overlap with those of meningitis, encephalitis, and near miss cot death.

The CT scan appearances are of a diffuse brain injury with bleeding into the subdural spaces and into the brain tissue (Fig 2.3). The features are commonly asymmetrical. The presence of cerebral oedema appears to take several hours to become detectable by CT scan. There is widespread neuronal damage, diffuse loss of blood supply to parts of the brain which evolve into low density areas, and, subsequently, cerebral atrophy.

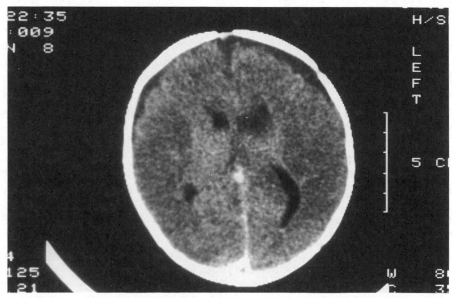

Fig 2.3   CT scan illustrating the shaken infant syndrome with diffuse brain injury and bleeding into the subdural spaces and brain tissue.

HYPOXIC ISCHAEMIC ENCEPHALOPATHY

Near-miss cot death

This is a diagnosis of exclusion in which an infant is laid down to sleep apparently well and is found moribund. The infant may have stopped breathing or have very inadequate respiratory effort and is either severely bradycardic (abnormally slow heart rate), or has undergone a cardiac arrest. The infant is resuscitated from this condition and the neurodevelopmental outcome is dependent on the duration of the hypoxia and ischaemia.

Aggressive resuscitation and intensive care management cannot reverse cell death consequent on the brain hypoxia and ischaemia.

Early indications of the severity of the hypoxic-ischaemic event are the severity of the metabolic acidosis, blood coagulation abnormalities, raised hepatic (liver) enzymes, and raised creatinine and urea. There is often an associated diarrhoea related to sloughing of the gastrointestinal mucosa.

The CT scan appearances following a severe hypoxic-ischaemic event are of cerebral oedema with loss of differentiation of the cortical grey and white matter and reduction in size of the cerebral ventricles. Subsequent scans show the evolution of areas of low density within the brain (Fig 2.4). There may be relative preservation of the blood supply to the cerebellum. The appearances are often symmetrical and there is no intracerebral bleeding.

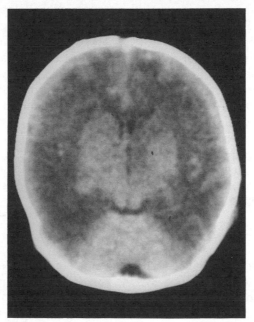

Fig 2.4 CT scan illustrating a severe hypoxic-ischaemic brain injury. There is low density throughout both cerebral hemispheres in comparison to the normal density of the cerebellum posteriorly.

Near drowning

The clinical features are similar to those described in the patient with the features of near miss cot death. The clinical outcome depends on the duration of hypoxia and ischaemia. The requirement for cardiopulmonary resuscitation and an initial pH of less than 7.0 are clinical indicators of a poor neurological outcome (Fandel and Bancalari, 1976). ICP monitoring and aggressive management of raised ICP do not affect the clinical outcome because the amount of cerebral oedema correlates with the severity of the hypoxic-ischaemic event.

'METABOLIC' AND INFECTIVE CONDITIONS CAUSING RAISED INTRACRANIAL PRESSURE

Reye's syndrome

This condition, of unknown aetiology, is characterized by vomiting, raised hepatic enzymes, raised plasma ammonia, fatty infiltration of the liver and other viscera (organs) and an acute, non-inflammatory encephalopathy with severe cerebral oedema. The hepatic failure is associated with disorders of coagulation, hypoglycaemia, lipid and amino acid metabolism. The neurological outcome correlates with the degree of coma and the most common cause of death is brainstem herniation syndrome secondary to marked cerebral oedema.

In some patients with Reye's syndrome, one of a group of inborn errors of metabolism has been detected and specific treatment of these has been associated with clinical improvement. An infectious triggering agent is thought to be a cause or contributory factor in some cases. Epidemiological studies have suggested that aspirin may also have an aetiological role in this condition. Since the recommendation that aspirin used as an antipyretic should be avoided in all children, very few cases have been notified in the UK (Brown *et al*, 1983).

Meningitis

Meningitis is associated with a purulent exudate over the meninges. This inflammation of cerebral blood vessels can cause infarction secondary to occlusion of blood vessels and interference with blood supply to areas of the brain. This may, in itself, cause cerebral oedema. In some cases, there is acute thrombosis of the venous blood sinuses which are involved in venous blood drainage from the brain. This obstruction to blood flow causes a catastrophic rise in ICP and is associated with the syndrome of acute brainstem herniation. In a group of children whose clinical state was such that they required intensive care management, ICP was elevated in all patients; and in those who died, this was associated with an inadequate CPP (Goitein and Tamir 1983).

Encephalitis

Encephalitis is an inflammation of the brain tissue itself. A viral aetiology is more likely but other infectious and toxic agents may be responsible. In a number of patients the aetiology is unknown. The nature and outcome of the acute brain injury relates to both the area of brain most severely affected, and the elevation of the ICP and the effect it has on the CPP.

CONCLUSION

The management of acute brain injury has four components; resuscitation, stabilization, investigation, and neuro-intensive care support. Outcome relates to the adequacy of clinical management and to the nature of the brain injury.

This chapter serves as an overview of the principles of management. Standard textbooks on paediatric intensive care will give additional detailed clinical information and more practical guidance.

REFERENCES

American Academy of Pediatrics. (1993). Shaken baby syndrome: inflicted cerebral trauma. *Pediatrics* **92**, 872–5.

Brown, A. K., Fikrig , S., and Finberg, L. (1983). Aspirin and Reye's syndrome. *Journal of Pediatrics* **102**, 157–8.

Fandel, I. and Bancalari, E. (1976). Near-drowning in children: clinical aspects. *Pediatrics* **58**, 573–9.

Goitein, K.J. and Tamir, I. (1983). Cerebral perfusion pressure in central nervous system infections of infancy and childhood. *Journal of Pediatrics* **103**, 40–3.

Jaspan, T., Narborough, G., Punt, J.A.G., and Lowe, J. (1992). Cerebral contusional tears as a marker of child abuse - detection by cranial sonography. *Pediatric Radiology*, **22**, 237–45.

Kalimo, H., Rehncrona, S., Soderfeldt, B., Olsson, Y., and Siesjo B.K. (1981). Brain lactic acidosis and ischemic cell damage. II. Histopathology. *Journal of Cerebral Blood Flow and Metabolism*, **1**, 313.

Muizelaar, J.P., Marmarou, A., Ward, J.D., *et al.* (1991). Adverse effects of prolonged hyperventilation in patients with severe head injury: a randomized clinical trial. *Journal of Neurosurgery*, **75**, 731–9.

Welch, K. (1980). The intracranial pressure in infants. *Journal of Neurosurgery*, **52**, 693–99.

3

Brain (head) injury team

Tony Baldwin, Julie Nash, and Richard Appleton

INTRODUCTION

Recovery from a brain injury is not like a recovery from any other injury, since the effects are far more complex and pervasive and affect a whole range of attributes. These changes can range from the subtle and barely noticed to being extremely significant and severe, fundamentally altering the child's emotional, intellectual, and social behaviour. They can be observed both in the acute stage, and frequently the deficits remain long past the point in which a total physical recovery has taken place. In some cases, skills have to be retaught and alternative strategies given, and the child's behaviour may need modifying. At the same time both the child and family need emotional support and reassurance.

Given the all-embracing range of problems that can follow an injury, no one professional group can provide all the relevant advice and support, and the emphasis therefore falls on a whole range of different professionals at different stages during the recovery process. The purpose of this chapter is to outline the philosophy, principles, and role of the multidisciplinary brain (head) injury rehabilitation team, and how it functions in our own hospital.

Brain-injury rehabilitation services for children have traditionally not been as well developed as those for adults, and it is only comparatively recently that it has become more widely recognized that the needs of neurologically impaired children differ from those of other children. There are possibly several reasons why this situation has developed, and as a group, head-injured children have been given a lower priority:

- firstly, there is a general belief that a child's brain is more resilient to injury than that of an adult; however, the converse is more likely to be true (Filley *et al.* 1887)
- there has been the persistent belief that the young and immature brain is more plastic; plasticity refers to the ability of intact areas of the brain to take over the function of the areas that have been damaged. However, many studies do not actually support this proposition and have shown that whereas some improvements and compensation can take place, subtle deficits may persist (Levin, *et al.* 1982; Levin and Benton 1986; Rutter 1982).

- it has to be noted that children, unlike adults, are neither in employment nor are they running a household or living independently; they are, by their very nature still being cared for by parents and do not incur the enormous financial costs in lost work, hospitalization, and care requirements of adults (Johnston and Hall 1994).

It is now widely accepted across the broad spectrum of services that children are not 'miniature adults', and that they require services in their own right which take account of their specific needs in a developmental context. Whereas the type and severity of head injuries may be similar in both children and adults, it must not be forgotten that the effects of these injuries may be quite different for a number of reasons, but predominantly because of the relative immaturity of the child's brain and the fact that the child is still in the early stages of the learning process. An adult has acquired the majority of the skills that he requires but children are still developing and are often only in the initial stages of acquiring the necessary skills. A child's head injury and subsequent rehabilitation therefore has to be considered in the light of the normal intellectual and physiological maturation which is taking place in the child who is still in his formative years of developing educational, social, and behavioural skills.

The development of services has also been hampered by the lack of long term follow-up; (Klonoff *et al* (1977) is one of the few studies that follows children up for a number of years. It is generally recognized that recovery does continue over quite a prolonged period of up to 5 years (Klonoff *et al.* 1977), but little is known as to how their recovery can be specifically aided during this period, although a number of rehabilitation approaches have been tried. Possibly one of the most worrying pictures has been painted by Wrightson *et al* (1995) whose study illustrated the effects that even quite mild head injuries can have on children. In this study children who had only very mild head injuries that did not necessarily involve loss of consciousness or admission to hospital during the pre-school period, were showing a delay in their educational attainments early in their school career.

THE NATURE OF THE PROBLEM

Whereas the child's return to the home environment has tremendous emotional advantages in providing a familiar and secure environment, it also has a disadvantage in that the services providing ongoing therapy are frequently fragmented. Local community services often lack the experience of working with any number of head-injured children by virtue of their low incidence within a given geographical area. The advantages of well co-ordinated community based services for adults was emphasised by Evans (1987), and of course the argument is even stronger for children whose life is even more community based.Most of the experience of the professionals who work with children who have been referred will be derived from working with children who have developmental problems, and therefore they may feel less confident in dealing with the wider issues that ensue from a child who has acquired difficulties.

Whereas the child's return home is initially met with relief by parents and child alike as it signifies medical stability and improvement and a welcome opportunity for the family to regain a degree of normality, family members may not be prepared to meet the changes that may have occurred; the emotional 'roller-coaster' that they experienced at the time of, and for the first few days and weeks after the accident, may start all over again. The child may not be the same child that left the home many weeks or months ago and a new individual may now have taken his place. The family has to readjust to a child who has a degree of disability and to cope with the uncertainty as to how this may affect the child in the long term (Wolkind and Rutter 1985).

The need for rehabilitation services for the head injured child has been recognised for a number of years and both the (British Paediatric Association and British Association of Paediatric Surgeons (BPA 1991) and the British Psychological Society (BPS 1989) have independently reported their concerns. The BPS has recently set up further working parties to examine the services for children and young adults who have acquired brain damage. The National Audit Office has also recommended the establishment of rehabilitation services for children and young people.

When a child first returns home, education may understandably have a low level of priority. However, this negates the very important role that education can and indeed has to, play in helping to rehabilitate the child. Within local education authorities there is no specific service or provision for head-or brain-injured children and therefore their needs are catered for within the context of a generic service. For pupils unable to go to school, tuition is provided at home, but this is often minimal and the child is usually provided with only a few hours of home teaching each week.

It is difficult to provide a systematic, planned procedure to allow the child to be reintegrated back into school. This usually happens as and when the child's parents feel that it is practical, and much depends on the attitude of the local school. In addition, there is often confusion as to how the child's needs should be met. The conflict between cognitive rehabilitation and education has been further exasperated by the rigidity imposed by the National Curriculum, which has placed great constraints and inflexibility on an overburdened school system.

Many head-injured children are fortunate to be able to return to their local mainstream school. Initially they are treated sympathetically, but this can quickly degenerate, particularly if the child does not have any obvious physical handicap. A physically competent child is assumed to be a normal child and therefore cognitive and behavioural difficulties are not always fully appreciated. The once able and possibly still intelligent child may see himself falling further and further behind in a competitive school environment. This does little for his self-esteem and soon a loss of self-confidence can spiral out of control. Difficulties with concentration and attention are frequently misunderstood and it may be assumed that the child is simply 'naughty' or has been spoilt following their accident.

Conflict between the child-centred rehabilitation personnel and a competitive school system is a very real possibility and it may be that the more individual approach cannot be easily achieved; we experience this when attempting to obtain extra resources for a head-injured child. Many Education Authorities have now adopted defined criteria which a child must meet before a Statement of Special Educational Need may be automatically considered e.g. more than three years reading delay at 10 years of age. Whereas this may be appropriate for a child who has developmental learning deficits, such policies cannot address the range of learning and behavioural difficulties which arise from acquired impairment where the problems can be much more subtle and pervasive. Unfortunately without a statement the child's needs have to be met from the school's own resources and these are usually already stretched to breaking point. The brain injured child may therefore not always be high on their list of priorities and much needed help cludes them even after much lobbying from the head injury team. Even if some limited help is secured it is difficult to find local personnel with the experience and expertise to address the child's complex range of difficulties. Not infrequently, children are unable to return to their mainstream school and have to receive some form of special education provision. For a child who once was performing well within a mainstream school, transfer into a special class or unit where other children have little appreciation of his needs can be problematic. The brain injured child will usually recall his ability to cope quite well within a mainstream setting and it can be extremely distressing for him to find that he is now in a class surrounded by children who, as he will perceive it, are less able, either mentally or physically. Although he will not be able to carry out his previous activities, he will recall having interest and success in them. His interests, therefore, can differ considerably from his new classmates. The nature of the learning disabilities of children who have developmental problems may show some similarities to children who have an acquired brain injury, but, frequently, the brain-injured child needs specific tuition and remedial programmes to address his specific underlying cognitive deficits, which are often not as obvious and easily recognized as for children who have developmental difficulties.

THE NEED FOR REHABILITATION SERVICES

Given the range of the head-injured child's difficulties, it is not surprising that many people working with head injured children believe that a coherent, multidisciplinary team approach is required. This was recognized by a working party of the British Paediatric Association and British Association of Paediatric Surgeons (BPA 1991). The growing evidence for the need of an interdisciplinary approach has been recognized for some time (Hall *et al* 1990) and attention has been drawn to the sometimes quite subtle, but still very significant, problems that can result from a head injury.

The need for rehabilitation services is now becoming generally recognized, possibly, in part, driven by the growth of specialist independent services that have developed in the United States. In recent years, in Great Britain, there has been development of a few specialist services that provide for the medium to long term; these are occasionally funded through insurance claims. However, the term 'rehabilitation' applied several years after the event is in this respect, rather misleading because it cannot make the child as he once was – something parents obviously wish for. Years after a head injury the child's difficulties need to be addressed as a learning disability with the appropriate techniques and methods aimed at improving functional skills rather than some attempt at returning the child to their pre-accident state. The fact that rehabilitation techniques even if only provided for a short period do help brain damaged patients was demonstrated by Ruff et al. [1987] and that rehabilitation intro-duced soon after a brain injury has occurred has come from both comparative animal work [Wall and Eggar 1971] and from looking at the long term efficacy of a formalized rehabilitation programme with adults [Mackay et al 1992]. It follows that rehabilitation programmes need a co-ordinated approach that follows some overall basic concept of the nature of the acquired disabilities and attempts to address them and of course obtain some functional outcome measures. Studies examining the efficacy of adult rehabilitation by Prigatano [1986] and Ben-Yishay et al [1988] have shown that improvements in functional coping skills, as demonstrated by increased rates of employability, were obtained from comprehensively planned and neuropsychologically derived programmes. However, even with these findings the development of adult rehabilitation services has been slow and clearly, with children, outcome measures are more difficult to identify and evaluate. The reasons for this are easy to follow in that faulty learning or behavioural difficulties can be dealt with before they have time to develop into significant and major problems, and, of course, the motivation and emotional reserves of the family can be channelled more positively. Difficulties can be anticipated before the child is placed in failure situations and an air of despondency and failure develops.

When working with brain-injured children we must remember that they are children first and foremost and have the emotional needs of all children, in particular, those of security and the necessity to re-establish parental contact and a degree of normality. In order to reassure parents, we feel that it is important that all those working with the child communicate freely, ensuring that a consistent message is given. Not uncommonly, parents may be given over-optimistic views by one particular professional only to have their hopes and expectations dashed when talking to another professional. It is therefore necessary that all those working with the child discuss the child's progress at regular intervals, highlighting areas of specific concern and prioritizing future approaches and changes in the rehabilitation programme. If parents do not receive meaningful feed back they may become over-pessimistic and feel that the professionals are hiding the truth. It is realistic not to expect to have all the answers to the questions posed by families. Many professionals may find this both a frustrating and a disturbing experience; it is therefore important for each professional involved with the child to be able to refer back to the whole team and not feel that they have to answer such questions alone.

HEAD INJURY REHABILITATION FOR CHILDREN

The head-injury rehabilitation team (known as the 'HIRT') at Alder Hey believes that effective provision of rehabilitation services has major implications or consequences on the recovery of children and their families, which may affect their long-term physical, intellectual, and emotional recovery. Furthermore, although the advances in emergency resuscitative treatment and improved neurosurgical facilities have resulted in a reduction in mortality, with this there has been a corresponding increase in the numbers of children who are surviving severe head injuries, who have major residual problems. Unfortunately, specialist rehabilitation services for these brain-injured children are very limited and have certainly not mirrored the increased and improved resuscitation and intensive-care services.

At present, most children who have suffered a moderate or severe head injury are either discharged from the neurosurgical ward or intensive-care unit to the referring hospital from where they were initially transferred or are discharged home to receive support from the general, community-based services. Unfortunately, neither may have the experience or resources (or both) to satisfactorily rehabilitate and support the children and families, thereby potentially limiting their potential recovery.

The head-injury team at Alder Hey developed out of the realization that what was needed was a multidisciplinary, coordinated, and systematic approach towards the management of the head-injured child in the early stages of recovery. Alder Hey serves a local (District) community as well as a larger (Regional) community; in addition, children may be referred from other health regions if it is felt that the service provided can aid the child's recovery, although obviously the distance of such a provision from the family's home has to be considered.

Regular head injury meetings are held weekly and are begun as soon as the child is placed on the head-injury register. They continue not only for the duration of the in-patient phase of the rehabilitation programme, but throughout the time of attendance as a day-patient for therapies or in the hospital school.

As anyone working within an institution will realize, there are many political and professional issues that arise when trying to establish an effective lay-management, multidisciplinary team. Departments may have their own agenda and list of priorities. The essential issue within the HIRT is to provide a focus of interdisciplinary working in order to ensure the greatest and holistic service to the child. It is therefore accepted as a necessary function of the team for the individuals to value and respect the expertise and experience of other members and to integrate alternative models and suggestions into their own, overall therapeutic, approach. In order to deliver an effective programme it is necessary for team members to accept a general accountability for the team and have a group or corporate (and obviously cooperative) identity within it. To work effectively this has to supersede their own departmental aims and goals. It is necessary that the individuals accept the trust and direction from outside their own department and realize how their own specific therapy objectives relate to the overall goals within the 'total' therapy programme.

CRITERIA FOR REFERRAL TO THE HEAD INJURY REHABILITATION TEAM

Children referred include all those who have been admitted to either the paediatric intensive care unit at the Royal Liverpool Children's Hospital or to the paediatric neurosurgical unit at Walton Hospital (Liverpool). Children who have suffered less severe injuries are referred to the HIRT (by surgeons under whom they are initially admitted), depending on their neurological status 24 hours after admission. In this latter group there is clearly a degree of flexibility. Each child who is referred will be assessed by a member of the neurology medical staff usually the consultant or senior registrar – who will then decide which children need to be formally 'accepted' and treated by the entire team. Potentially, this can lead to a large number of children who would benefit from rehabilitation; but given the limited resources available, priorities have to be set.

More recently, children from outside the Mersey region, or those who have suffered head injuries some weeks or even months earlier, have also been admitted to the programme if it is felt that their specific needs can best be dealt with by the specific expertise of the team. The team also accepts for inclusion those who have suffered a non-traumatic (atraumatic) brain injury such as a hypoxic or ischaemic cerebral insult (following a prolonged cardiac arrest, stroke or encephalitis). The rationale for this is that, obviously, many of the problems, needs, and methods of rehabilitation in these children are similar to those who have suffered traumatic brain ('head') injuries.

The criteria for admission of children onto the head injury rehabilitation team programme is based primarily on the severity of the child's problems, recognizing the strong link between the severity of the head injury and the probable long-term effects and functional outcome (Knights *et al.* 1991). Given the large number of children who could potentially benefit from the programme, some children are, unfortunately, not able to be accepted. There are many children who have suffered minor or even mild head injuries who, based on the initial neurological assessment, are felt not to require 'formal' rehabilitation. However, this does not mean that various members of the head-injury team are not dealing with the child in their general professional capacity; i.e. the child may be receiving physiotherapy or being reviewed by the neurologist because of seizures. In addition, the child may be initially difficult to assess, particularly if he has fractured limbs or other major injuries. It may be that as soon as a formal neurological assessment has been possible, the child is then introduced to, and enrolled with, the rest of the rehabilitation team.

PRE-BRAIN INJURY INFORMATION

An important aspect of recovery is often that of knowing what the child was like before the injury. A number of studies (Brown *et al* 1981; Hass *et al* 1987 Klonoff 1971) have shown that many children who sustain a head injury had some pre-existing learning or behavioural problems (or both), although at least one other study (Donders 1992) has not shown any pre-morbid problems.

Most studies have also indicated that the head-injured child is most likely to come from lower socio-economic groupings and be associated with poorer housing conditions. Their fathers are more likely to be unemployed and parents are more likely to be divorced or separated. As one may appreciate, these conditions are generally to be found within inner-city areas and the housing estates of our larger cities. It follows that it is often this group of families that have the least emotional or physical resources to assist with the rehabilitation of the head injured child. As Chadwick *et al* (1981))found, head-injured children tended to have lower IQs and lower school attainments than their controls. From our own experiences, a total of 71% of children referred to the team with a head injury had pre-existing problems: 42% had learning and behavioural difficulties, 11% had behavioural difficulties alone, and 18% just learning difficulties. When the nature of their behavioural difficulties was looked at more closely, 55% had attentional difficulties, 20% had attentional and coordination difficulties, and 25% displayed attentional and antisocial behaviours. No children had just coordination difficulties or antisocial behaviour.

The nature of the injury and how it was sustained appears to be a relevant factor as our results showed that 38% of children involved in a road traffic accident and 71% of those involved in a fall, had pre-existing problems. It is difficult – and perhaps erroneous – to make a direct relationship, but it follows that the child who had poor attentional skills or was impulsive prior to the head injury may have put himself more seriously at risk. Alternatively, the child may have had some general or specific learning difficulties prior to the accident and these difficulties may therefore be confused with apparent deficits resulting from the accident, although from experience we have to conclude that any head injury often (and not surprisingly), appears to exaggerate any pre-existing deficits.

As an essential function of the team we therefore ask for pre-injury information as soon as possible. When children are admitted to the ward their parents' permission is sought for us to request such information from the schools. The hospital school sends a questionnaire to the school and makes contacts, in order to inform them of the situation and explain the need for such information. This helps us to understand the child more fully, and therefore helps in all future discussions with the child and his parents as it places remarks and problems in context. It also has the advantage of making a very important link with the child's school and teacher, and helps to reassure them that making contact with the child would be helpful as sometimes schools may feel a little unsure as to whether they are intruding on parents' anxieties. At this stage we feel that the situation is too emotive to ask the child's parents about his pre-injury behaviour pattern, and so this information is sought later.

WHO IS IN THE TEAM?

The head injury team comprises the family and those professional staff who commonly work with the head-injured child. This includes members of the ward nursing staff, therapists, and medical staff. As the child's rehabilitation programme proceeds, and, of course, depending upon the child's recovery and the needs of his parents, the hospital schoolteachers and psychologists (clinical and educational) may also become involved. The involvement of each professional group, and the specific contributions that they are able to make, may obviously alter, depending upon the child's place in the rehabilitation process. In order that parents are familiar with the various professions referred to, they are given a head-injury booklet which outlines the role of individual professions and the nature of their work.

Hospital doctor

When a child is initially admitted to the hospital it is the accident and emergency (casualty) staff who will attend to the child and assess his condition. If the child is unconscious or has breathing difficulties, experiences seizures, or is seriously ill, then he is usually admitted to the intensive care unit. On the intensive care unit the medical and nursing staff will monitor the child's progress. When the child is sufficiently recovered and stable he is transferred to the neurology ward, where he remains until discharge from the in-patient phase of the rehabilitation programme. On the neurology ward, the child's care is supervised by the consultant paediatric neurologist, with involvement from the other specialist services as and when necessary, including neurosurgery, ophthalmology, and orthopaedics.

The duration of the in-patient phase is dependent upon many factors but is largely based on the child's nursing and medical needs. When these can be appropriately seen to by his parents, and they are confident and comfortable in his management, the child can be discharged back to the security and familiarity of his own home.

Nursing staff

When a child is admitted to any ward it is general policy to have a named staff member who is responsible for him and to whom the parents and child can relate. The nurses on the specialist neurology ward where most of the children's rehabilitation takes place, do not wear uniforms. The reason for this is that nursing on the ward is centred around the family and it is important that the child is not 'put off', or the family intimidated, by a uniform. Nurses do wear name badges in order that they are readily recognized by children and parents alike. They are always available to answer parents' questions and concerns and help the child while he is on the ward, being a common person to whom the child and parent can turn to. Chapter 4 discusses the work of the nursing staff in detail.

Play therapists

The play therapist's role on the HIRT is to provide for the social and emotional well-being of the child. They are also able to provide comforting care and support to the child when it may not be possible for the parents to be in attendance. Within the HIRT team the play therapists initiate a head-injury progress chart for parents so that they can take an active part in checking their child's progress and needs in all areas of the rehabilitation programme. They are also vital in helping to prepare the child for any further tests that may be needed, using simple explanations, photographs, or toys, rather than allowing him to develop unnecessary anxiety and misunderstanding.

Social worker

The social worker's role on the rehabilitation team is to offer support to the parents at any time during admission, and also to provide that vital link for when the patient goes home. Social-work involvement often begins at the time of admission or certainly at the time of transfer to the neurology ward. The social worker is able to offer advice on welfare and other financial benefits, advise on where and how to seek other support and make arrangements for other children to be looked after to allow the parents more time to spend with the child in hospital. They are also able to help in cases where parents are in employment and may need to request absence, and will also liaise with outside agencies in order to help arrange adaptations and equipment for when the child returns home.

Psychologists

Following a head injury, both family and child suffer major upheavals in their lives. The family will have gone through a tremendously stressful experience and often suffer emotional difficulties, along with the child who may be suffering behavioural and mood changes. He may have lost some of the skills he had previously learnt, and in some cases may find difficulties learning new skills. Other members within the extended family will also have been affected, particularly brothers and sisters.

The psychologists, both clinical and educational, help in the assessment of the child's individual needs and provide ongoing support, particularly when liaising with local services in order to ensure that the child and his family receive the appropriate level of support and provision for when he comes to leave the hospital.

Community doctor

The community paediatrician is able to help arrange appointments for the child to be seen by the local health clinic and ensure that their local, paramedical, community support services are in place. Following discharge from the in-patient phase of the programme, children frequently return to the hospital at regular intervals for out-patient appointments; although some of the medical cover is passed over to the local community paediatrician who can liaise with the relevant local education authority (LEA) in order to arrange specialist provision. The community paediatrician is usually the most appropriate doctor to ensure that all the child's various needs – medical and other – are adequately addressed following discharge from hospital, even though there may still be continuing 'specialist' medical input.

Speeech and language therapist

Speech and language therapists have an important role to play in the management of both feeding and communication problems in the brain injured child. The type and frequency of any intervention will vary depending on the needs of the individual child. However, the speech and language therapist should become involved once the child is reasonably stable and having periods of wakefulness. Initially, assessment of the child's ability to swallow safely will be required so that he can be weaned from tube-feeding back to oral-feeding as soon as it is safe to do so. Some children will need help to regain control of movements of the mouth, as well as to coordinate breathing and swallowing. The speech and language therapist will also, in conjunction with the occupational therapists and physiotherapists, advise on appropriate positioning of the child for feeding as well as establishing the utensils required and the type and consistency of foods appropriate, until full oral feeding has been re-established. The role and function of the speech and language therapist is discussed in more detail in Chapter 7.

Occupational therapist

The role of the occupational therapist is to assist the child to regain maximum independence following the injury. The main areas that are covered are fine motor skills, broad perceptual ability, and self help-skills. They are instrumental in assisting children to regain those crucial functional skills that will enable them to care for themselves and continue to regain or develop their independence. Specific support continues for much of the child's stay in hospital and then, frequently, into the out-patient phase of rehabilitation, with advice and support being given to the child's parents and teachers. There is a clear overlap and many shared areas of treatment with the physiotherapist, as discussed in Chapter 5.

Physiotherapist

The physiotherapist is usually the first therapist to start actively working with the child, frequently beginning on the intensive-care unit with chest care and advice on appropriate changes of position and possible splinting to prevent joint contractures. Therapy at the initial stages of recovery involves the active movement and manipulation of the child to prevent abnormal postures and motor patterns and promote normal sensory and motor development. Their involvement will usually continue throughout a child's rehabilitation programme if the child has continuing motor, whether tone or movement, difficulties. Continuing physiotherapy will be transferred to the community services if long term treatment is required. Hydrotherapy is incorporated in most of the physiotherapy programmes.

Teachers

Each brain-injured child is assigned to a class teacher in the appropriate age range. One of these teachers acts as a 'link' teacher, to provide important links between the hospital school and the child's previous school. This is particularly relevant if and when the child returns to his previous school in a gradual and stepwise fashion. The child's class teacher works with the other teachers and the relevant support staff in the hospital in delivering the child's individual education plan (IEP).

The headteacher of the hospital school is responsible for admissions to the school. In most situations, the headteacher or link teacher arranges a preliminary visit for the child and his parents at a time that is convenient for the relevant class teacher, and, if possible, accompanies the child on this visit.

TEAM MEETINGS

Weekly interdisciplinary team meetings are held at which each child is discussed, whether he is an in-patient or day-patient attending the hospital school. The meetings are chaired by the community paediatrician, or in her absence, by the paediatric neurologist. The decision was made that the community paediatrician has the administrative role, as the named person within the health service with the legal responsibility of liaising and notifying local authorities as to the essential specific needs of individual children, as suggested in the report by the BPA Working Party (BPA 1991).

Newly registered children, together with all other children being treated, are discussed with team members at the head injury meeting. A medical update is given on each child and team members discuss any significant changes in their own particular areas. Discussion takes place on future aims of treatment and members gain valuable information from other disciplines. It is essential that all team members work and communicate together, throughout each child's rehabilitation, constantly re-evaluating their needs, redefining objectives and adapting the rehabilitation programme depending upon each child's progress.

Decisions are made as to the significance of various aspects of their rehabilitation and the way those aspects should be addressed. Potential problems are also highlighted, discussed and appropriate solutions are proposed and implemented if considered relevant. Comments from the child's parents and if possible, the child himself, are also welcomed as they are important contributors to the overall programme.

The meeting operates as an open forum, with all members of the team able to assimilate information offered by one member and therefore integrate key elements into their own specific programme if necessary. Decisions are made on a group basis with the community paediatrician and consultant neurologist taking responsibility for the medical supervision of the child, although the person who is acting as the co-ordinator for a particular child may be any one of the various professionals involved. This process ensures that the family and child receive one cogent overall description of the child's level of functioning within the total programme, rather than several individual accounts which are often diverse, and can be fragmented, redundant and subsequently confusing to the parents.

If the child's parents cannot be present at the team meetings, someone will take responsibility for talking to them about how their child's rehabilitation is proceeding and informing them of any decisions that may relate to his future therapies or need for continued attendance at the hospital school or, indeed, discharge from the rehabilitation programme. This feedback is of crucial importance; parents may become understandably concerned and pessimistic about their child's progress, and feel as though the truth is being hid from them if they are not kept informed. Of course any decisions are made with the parents agreement; and if parents are unsure as to the need for changes in the present regime, they are fully involved in any discussions and decisions. Not surprisingly, parents have many questions which need to be answered. These are often asked of all the different professionals involved, with, consequently, conflicting answers, which is frustrating to both team members and parents alike. It is therefore important for each professional involved with the child to refer questions back to the team meetings and not feel that they have to answer the questions alone.

As well as the weekly meetings which are attended by all the team members, meetings take place between individuals to discuss specific management issues and plans These commonly include the:

- link teacher and therapists (usually the occupational, speech, and physiotherapist)

- physio and occupational therapists
- play therapists and the other therapists
- teachers and the psychologists.

TEAMWORK

It is unfortunate that there is very little information available as to the effectiveness of different rehabilitation models. As Johnston and Hall (1994) concluded, there is a need for a more systematic collection of compatible data that can be used across studies, in order that different programmes can be evaluated. This is becoming particularly necessary in the days where outcomes are looked at by managers and where the cost-effectiveness of any service and treatment model is always being considered – now termed 'evidence based medicine'. Unfortunately, working with individuals we are generally in a situation of evaluating the effectiveness of rehabilitation based on single cases, who may or may not have recovered solely through their own efforts and that of their family and independently of any formal rehabilitation programme. However, there is evidence to suggest that rehabilitation introduced early is more beneficial and effective than if begun later (MacKay *et al.* 1992).

There are no formal data demonstrating that recovery from brain injuries is greater if rehabilitation services are coordinated and multidisciplinary rather than individual and fragmented; however, it is instinctively more likely that a multidisciplinary-team approach would be more effective. Even though there is little direct evidence available to prove that it is superior, we feel that the main value is in providing a comprehensive and cogent model of stability and care to the individual. The Alder Hey team therefore operates this multidisciplinary approach and model of delivery, with each discipline working with the patient using its own professional expertise, but in such a way that there is always open and regular discussion between the professionals, thus maintaining some continuity. However, there is clearly an inherent danger in this approach. It is easy for the different professionals from diverse disciplines to fail to integrate each therapy into an overall cogent model, and there is a very real danger that different approaches may be used with the same child (i.e. different use of language, different expectancies of what the child can or cannot understand).

The HIRT did consider an interdisciplinary team-model approach, which has been proposed as being more efficient and effective. In this approach, one member of the team carries out the basic programme, regardless of their own professional training or background. The scheme is not dissimilar to the concept of using conductors, so favoured by the Peto method of teaching. However, the comprehensive team approach has never been appropriately proven. The team therefore considered the use of a primary therapist or key worker when working with the child. They felt that it would not be possible to deliver and maintain the high level of individualized expertise and support for the child. In addition, a key therapist who is not a specialist within their own right would not be sensitive to the improvements or difficulties that an individual child may be showing and would therefore not be aware of the often subtle changes that can occur during recovery.

There is obviously a need for a consistent and coordinated, if not fully orchestrated, approach with all the therapies for the brain-injured child. It is therefore extremely important that members use similar interactive styles, behavioural techniques, and management strategies when working with the child. The aim of the rehabilitation process is to help highlight the underlying deficits and provide the child with alternative strategies and coping mechanisms that he will be able to use in his normal environment. In many respects this is similar to the information-processing model of cognition, taking into account the neuropsychological models that are currently being hypothesized. If a child's difficulties are addressed in the early stages, the behaviour problems that not uncommonly follow a brain injury may be alleviated, which may at least establish a more stable basis for the potential recovery and successful return of the child into his community and peer group.

MAINTAINING THE GRADIENT

One of the most essential features that we have found of importance in rehabilitating children is trying to maintain a gradient. It is beneficial to both parents and child to feel that there is a gradual road to recovery. Without promises, one is trying to maintain a concept of progress, no matter how small, and gradually through this progress one can start to provide some indications as to the long-term effects. Possibly for the first time in their lives, parents have to be introduced to the concept that a child's progress can be slow and steps may be exceedingly small. This may be something that is all too familiar to parents with a disabled child, but for parents who have seen their child grow up quite normally and taken for granted the acquisition of new skills, the realization that the skills now have to be taught and progress may be exceedingly slow is usually a very hard concept to accept. However, if it is not accepted with a positive attitude and approach, it can lead both parents and child into a rapidly spiralling cycle of despair and despondency. As with most aspects of life, keeping a positive attitude is one of the most crucial features of healthy living; it is important that the team have this attitude but without being overly optimistic or expressing unrealistic expectations.

Finally, and understandably, parents and other family members not infrequently experience anger and frustration which may be directed against any or all of the professionals involved with their child, the person who may have caused the accident which resulted in the head injury, or themselves. Clearly, this anger and frustration must be addressed as it could adversely affect their child's recovery and the effectiveness of the rehabilitation programme (Gans 1983; McMordie *et al.* 1991). The team has developed its own education and 'self-support' programme in an attempt to cope with the increasing workload (and increasing severity of some of the brain-injured children), and its inherent demands and stresses (McLaughlin and Carey 1993 McLaughlin and Erdman 1992). However, it has to be appreciated that professional development on its own may not necessarily help resolve the emotional stresses (Schlenz *et al* 1995) and in this respect a supportive team approach can help both 'client' and colleague.

REFERENCES

Ben-Yishay, Y., Silver, S. M., Paisetsky, E. and Rattock, J. (1987). Vocational outcome after intensive holistic cognitive rehabilitation. Journal of Head Trauma Rehabilitation, **2**, 35–45.

British Paediatric Association and British Association of Paediatric Surgeons. (1991). *Report of a Working Party: Guidelines on the management of head injuries in childhood.* BPA, London.

British Psychological Society. (1989). *Services for young patients with acquired brain damage.* British Psychological Society, St. Andrew's House, Leicester.

Brown, G., Chadwick, O., Shaffer, D., Rutter, M., and Traub, M. (1981). A prospective study of children with head injuries. III. Psychiatric sequelae. *Psychological Medicine*, **11**, 63–78.

Chadwick, O., Rutter, M., Shaffer, D. and Shrout, P. (1981). A study of children with head injuries. IV. Specific cognitive deficits. *Journal of Clinical and Experimental Neuropsychology*, **3**, 101–20.

Donders, J. (1992). Pre-morbid behavioural and psychological adjustment in children with traumatic brain injury. *Journal of Abnormal Child Psychology*, **20**, 233–46.

Evans, C.D. (1987). Rehbilitation of head injury in a rural community. *Clinical Rehabilitation*, **1**, 133–7.

Filley, C.M., Lee, D., Cranberg, M.D., Alexander, M.P., and Hart, E.J. (1987). Neurobehavioural outcome after a closed head injury in childhood and adolescence. *Archives of Neurology*, **44**, 194–8.

Gans, J. S. (1983). Hate in the rehabilitation setting. *Archives of Physical Medicine and Rehabilitation*, **64**, 176–9.

Gurdjian, E.S. and Webster, J.E. (1958). *Head injuries: medicine, diagnosis, and management.* Little, Brown & Co., Boston.

Hall, D.M., Johnson, S.L., and Middleton, J. (1990). Rehabilitation of head-injured children. *Archives of Disease in Childhood*, **65**, 553–6.

Hass, J., Cope, D.N., and Hall, K. (1987). Pre-morbid prevalance of poor acedemic performance in severe head injury. *Journal of Neurology, Neurosurgery, and Psychiatry*, **50**, 52–6.

Johnston, M.V., Hall, K.M. (1994). Outcomes evaluation in TBI Rehabilitation. Part 1: Overview and system principles. *Archives of Physical Medicine and Rehabilitation*, **75**, SC1-SC9.

Klonoff, H., Low, M.D., and Clark, C. (1977). Head injuries in children. A prospective five-year follow-up. *Journal of Neurology, Neurosurgery, and Psychiatry*, **40**, 1211–19.

Klonoff, H. (1971). Head injuries in children. Predisposing factors, accident conditions, accident proneness and sequelae. *American Journal of Public Health*, **61**, 2405–17.

Knights, R.M., Ivan, L.P., Ventureyra, E.C.G., Benturologo, C., Stobbart, C., Winogron, W., and Bawden, H.N. (1991). The effects of head injury in children on neuropsychological and behavioural functioning. *Brain Injury*, **5**, 339–51.

Levin, H.S., and Benton, A.L. (1986). Developmental and aquired dyscalculia in children. In *Child development and learning behaviour*, (ed. I. Flehmig and L.Stern), Gustav Fisher, Stuttgart.

Levin, H.S., Benton, A.L., and Grossman, R.G. (1982). *Neurobehavioural consequences of closed head injury*. Oxford University Press, New York.

McLaughlin, A.M. and Erdman, J. (1992). Rehabilitation staff stress as it relates to patient acuity and diagnosis. *Brain Injury*, **6**, 59-64.

McLaughlin, A.M. and Carey, J.L. (1993). The adversarial alliance: developing therapeutic relationships between families and the team in brain injury rehabilitation. *Brain Injury*, **7**, 45-51.

McMordie, W.R., Rogers, K.F., and Barker, S.L. (1991). Consumer satisfaction with services provided to head-injured patients and their families. *Brain Injury*, **5**, 43-51.

MacKay, L.E., Bernstein B.A., Chapman, P.E., Morgan, A.S., and Milazzo, L.S. (1992). Early intervention in severe head injury: long-term benefits of a formalized program. *Archives of Physical Medicine and Rehabilitation*, **73**, 635–41.

Medical Disability Society. (1988). *The management of traumatic brain injury*. Medical Disability Society, London.

National Curriculum. (1995). DFE, Crown Publication HMSO.

Oddy, M., Bonham, E., McMillan, T., Stroud, A., and Rickard, S. (1989). A comprehensive service for the rehabilitation and long-term care of head injury survivors. *Clinical Rehabilitation*, **3**, 253–9.

Ponsford, J, (1995). *Traumatic brain injury: rehabilitation for everyday adaptive living*. Lawrence Erlbaum Associates Ltd. Hove.

Prigatano, G. P. (1986). *Neuropsychological rehabilitation after brain injury*. John Hopkins University Press, Baltimore.

Ruff, R., Baser, C., Klein, T. *et al.* (1987). Neuropsychological rehabilitation: an experimental study with head-injured patients. *Journal of Clinical and Experimental Neuropsychology*, **9**, 5–12.

Rutter, M. (1982) Developmental neuropsychiatry: issues and prospects. *Journal of Clinical Neuropsychology*, **4**, 91-115.

Schlenz, K. G., Guthrie, M. R., and Dudgeon, B. (1995). Burnout in occupational therapists and physical therapists working in head injury rehabilitation. *American Journal of Occupational Therapy*, **49**, 986–93.

The Education of Sick Children DFE and NHS. (1994) Joint Circular, (12/94), 60-3.

Wall, P.D. and Egger, M.D. (1971). Formation of new connections in adult rat brains after partial differentiation. *Nature*, **232**, 542–5.

Wolkind, S. and Rutter, M. (1985). Separation, loss and family relationships. In *Child & adolescent psychiatry* (2nd ed), (ed. M. Rutter and C. Herson), pp. 34-57. Blackwell Scientific Publications, Oxford.

Wrightson, P., McGinn, V. and Gronwall, D. (1995). Mild head injury in preschool children: evidence that it can be associated with a persisting cognitive defect. *Journal of Neurology, Neurosurgery, and Psychiatry*, **59**, 375–80.

4

Immediate medical and nursing needs

Julie Nash, Richard Appleton, Bridget Rowland,
Jane Saltmarsh and Julie Sellars

The purpose of this chapter is to identify and discuss the more common
immediate nursing and medical issues, and needs of the brain-injured child
(and his family), following the acute resuscitation period and on transfer to
the neuro-rehabilitation ward. The chapter also outlines and discusses the
importance of play as an integral component of the rehabilitation process.

TRANSITION TO REHABILITATION

The initial period of rehabilitation takes place while the child is an in-patient,
occasionally on the intensive care or neurosurgical unit, but more commonly
on the neurology ward. The child is transferred to the neurology ward from
the paediatric intensive care unit, the paediatric neurosurgical unit at Walton
Hospital in Liverpool, or from other hospitals (regionally or nationally) via a
referral to the head injury rehabilitation team (HIRT).

The transition from intensive care to rehabilitation ward can be a traumatic
and confusing time for the parents and the child. Leaving behind a high-tech
environment, with its monitors and reassuring numbers of staff, to arrive on a
busy, often noisy, neurology ward can be understandably difficult. To assist
in improving this transition, the primary nurse and play specialist will visit
the child and family whilst still on the intensive care or neurosurgical unit, to
introduce themselves and to arrange a time for the parents to visit the
neurology ward prior to the child's transfer. This ensures that the parents
know who will be caring for their child and the environment in which that
care will be given. Discussion focuses on many issues, including:

- what to expect when their child (and themselves) are transferred to the
  neurology ward
  - the environment
  - the nursing staff
  - the other members of the team who will become involved with the
    rehabilitation programme
  - that the doctors may arrange some investigations (e.g. a CT or MRI brain
    scan or EEG) or request special assessments, including tests of swallow-
    ing, sight, and hearing etc.

- the possible emotional or behavioural problems that the children may experience as a result of the transfer
- the fact that, particularly if the brain injury was severe, the child may behave and function very much like a newborn infant, and because of this he will have to be taught – and learn – many of the basic skills all over again (e.g. toileting, washing, dressing, and eating).
- a very general idea of the likely duration of in-patient rehabilitation, although this is clearly very difficult as each child is different and will depend upon a number of factors, including the severity of the brain and other injuries, and the child's usual place of residence. (Nevertheless, this is, understandably, one of the most common questions asked of the HIRT members by the parents when their child is transferred.)

These discussions are invariably repeated once the child has actually been transferred as parents frequently forget much of what they have been told or heard in the emotional chaos of either the intensive care or neurosurgical units. Parents and families are also given a booklet which explains the purpose of the HIRT and the roles of each of the team members as a written reminder of, and reinforcement to, these initial discussions. The final page of this booklet includes some general points of advice:

- do ask, no matter how simple or trivial you may think the question might be
- do visit as often as you want – and bring other members of the family or your child's friends
- don't forget that other family members (particularly your other children) need you too . . . Brothers and sisters may actually help your child to recover more quickly
- don't forget to eat and sleep to keep up your strength. You will need your strength to look after your child – and the rest of the family
- don't be surprised if you feel angry towards the staff. This is all part of the shock and the pain you have gone through – we understand this
- don't ever lose hope.

Many parents believe that once their child wakes up they will soon be back to normal. Whilst obviously remaining optimistic about the future it is important to be realistic and honest – and importantly – to answer their questions as fully and as truthfully (and often repeatedly) as is possible.

FAMILY-CENTRED CARE

The philosophy of our unit is that of a partnership with parents in caring for their child. The family has been identified as one of the most important variables in determining the outcome of care. Therefore to include the family actively from the moment that the child is being treated will hopefully enhance and increase the beginning, and subsequent rate of, recovery (Dittmar 1989).

The staff on the neurology ward do not wear uniforms because they wish to promote a friendly, non-threatening environment for the child to assist in the transition from intensive care to rehabilitation nursing. The no-uniform policy was established following consultation with parents, children, and their families as well as nursing and medical staff on the unit in 1991. As rehabilitation can be a lengthy process, the ward understandably becomes the child's temporary home; and as they become more aware of their surroundings they are less intimidated by the nursing staff wearing 'normal' clothes, and a relationship built on friendship and trust is developed. As is the rule in most children's units or hospitals, medical staff do not wear white coats; this encourages the perception by both parents and children that the doctors are more 'approachable' and friendly, without losing any respect.

The nurses work in two teams: the 'Winnies' wear green T-shirts and the 'Tiggers' yellow T-shirts. Prior to admission, the child is allocated a primary or named nurse who works within one of the teams. Thus, if the child's own nurse is not on duty then they know that another nurse within their team will look after them. All staff and members of the HIRT wear name badges and all are introduced to the child and family, as the team is fully aware that its members must be readily identifiable for the parents and their child.

It is often far easier for nurses to assume total care for the child, but by encouraging the parents to be actively involved this will reduce their sense of helplessness and build up their confidence in the care of their child. The parents' sense of anxiety and incapacity to protect their child frequently leads to a sense of powerlessness. The importance of encouraging and allowing parents and significant others to be involved in the care of the child cannot be overemphazised – it facilitates the parents regaining some control over their child's care, thereby removing and dispelling some of their feelings of helplessness and frustration which they may have experienced in the intensive care unit (Calef 1959).

Involvement in the care of the child is extended to include grandparents, siblings and others who may have been closely involved with the child (e.g. a child-minder or nanny), which increases their understanding and acceptance of any disabilities and assists in planning realistic long term goals. This continuing involvement helps to preserve the health of the family unit and increases the security of the brain injured child. Upon transfer to the ward it is important to be aware of the parents' concerns and apprehensions. It is crucial that on the day of, and during the first few days following, transfer their trust is gained and a successful rapport developed to encourage an effective staff/parental relationship; this also applies to the staff/child relationship, although clearly this may take somewhat longer to establish, depending on the severity of the child's brain injury and their 'awareness'.

In this relaxed and friendly environment, family-centered care can flourish. Time must be allowed for a settling in period for the child and family. It is important that the parents do have time to spend with their other children and to return home; as they become more confident in their child's recovery they usually feel more able to do this.

THE ROLE OF THE NURSE AND PLAY SPECIALIST

'The unique function of the nurse is to assist the individual, sick or well, in the performance of those activities contributing to health or its recovery (or to a peaceful death) that he would perform unaided if he had the necessary strength, will, or knowledge. And to do this in such a way as to help him gain independence as rapidly as possible.' (Henderson 1966).

Nurses who plan the care for the brain injured child are in a unique and crucial position: they are the only discipline in the HIRT's rehabilitation programme to incorporate a 24-hour time span for their planned nursing intervention. Nurses are of particular importance in brain injury rehabilitation because they are the only staff routinely present in the evenings, throughout the night, at every meal and at weekends (Appleton 1994: Davidson 1989). This is also true for parents – which is why they are considered a vital part of the team.

The role of the play staff is to stimulate the child and provide for the child's social and emotional well-being and to support the parents while the child is an in-patient. The play specialist and nursing staff attend the weekly HIRT meetings, providing opportunities to liaise with all therapists and to identify key problems.

The nursing staff, in conjunction with the play staff, are the pivotal members of the head-injury team at the time of and for the first few days (occasionally weeks) after the child has been transferred, and are the springboard for the successful initiation of the rehabilitation programme. They are also the common denominator throughout the entire in-patient period of the programme. By updating and informing other members of the team about the child's progress, the nursing and medical team-members can ensure that the therapists become involved in the child's rehabilitation at the appropriate time. In addition, it is often the nurses (and not the doctors) who are first approached by parents over certain specific medical issues – which may then be brought to the attention of the medical staff.

The most important things that a nurse can give a brain-injured child and their family are understanding, time, and patience, whilst promoting an environment in which confidence can be gained, new skills learnt, and the child can be assisted to realize their recovery potential.

ASSESSMENT (INITIAL AND ONGOING)

In the initial stages, the first concern is ensuring the child's safety, particularly if he is unconscious. The subsequent rehabilitation and its planning must commence with an assessment of the child. The purpose of the assessment is important in determining the child's state of health, mental state, and lifestyle before the injury (the pre-morbid state), e.g.:

- the child's developmental stage
- if the child had any significant disability or medical condition
- what sort of vocabulary the child had, and if he speaks and understands English
- who the child related well (and best) to prior to the injury

Talking to the parents and family builds up a picture of the child's personality prior to the injury and is important in determining the most appropriate initial approach to the individual child's rehabilitation programme.

An additional purpose of the initial assessment is to assess the child's and family's needs at this moment in time to enable the primary nurse to negotiate a plan of care with the parents. The assessment tool we use is adapted from Roper *et al.*'s 'activities of daily living' model (Roper *et al.* 1983).

Obviously some of the children admitted into the HIRT programme will be unconscious whilst others will be more aware and orientated, depending on the severity of the injury and the length of time since the injury. The following provides a brief summary of the main areas which must be addressed by the nursing (and medical) staff during their initial and ongoing assessment of each child.

Breathing

- Duration of ventilatory support and length of time since extubated
- Does the child have a tracheostomy (size and type of tube and the date of the last tube change) and how frequently suction is required.
- Is the child experiencing any respiratory difficulties; does he require oxygen; is there any indication to monitor the child's oxygen saturation transcutaneously?
- Does the child require chest physiotherapy or suction (emphazising close liaison with the physiotherapist)?

- Does the child have any pre-existing respiratory problem (e.g. asthma) and are the child's usual appropriate medications being prescribed?

If the child is likely to need a tracheostomy for weeks or months, then a training programme will need to be provided for both the parents and other relevant carers. The timing of this training will clearly depend on individual families and how able they feel to cope with learning new skills. There may be associated needs for training carers (for tracheostomy care) in school. Although this may seem to be a long way ahead, from our experience the earlier it is identified that a carer is required for the child to attend school the better, as this specific resource issue needs to be addressed by the health authority and local education authority, which may take some time.

Sleeping

What was the childs sleep pattern like before the brain injury; is he a light or deep sleeper; do noises wake him easily? (If, so then consider where in the ward or unit he can be most appropriately nursed. If a single room is needed, it is important to consider his needs for socialization when making this decision.)

- Does he normally sleep in a bed or a cot?
- Does he normally share a room with siblings?
- Does he like a light on overnight?
- Any soother or favourite toy that he takes to bed with him.
- What is his current pattern of sleep?

Children recovering from a brain injury tire very quickly and this must be taken into account when planning the child's rehabilitation programme. In the early and intermediate stages of the programme there must be adequate periods of rest and sleep between the different therapy sessions. In the immediate post-transfer period the child may be very irritable and restless and a period of night sedation may help to re-establish a good sleep pattern and reduce day time drowsiness which may otherwise adversely affect a child's response to his rehabilitation programme and short-term recovery. Some of the drugs which are most commonly used by the team include short-acting benzodiazepines, chloral hydrate and melatonin (for sleep disturbance), and amantadine, chlorpromazine and buspirone (for marked irritability and agitation). The use of these drugs is reviewed every couple of days and their continued prescription is determined by the child's needs and response.

The nursing staff and therapists will timetable the therapies to allow the child to have rest periods through the day. Initially, the child will only manage a couple of therapy sessions a day without tiring; if he is too tired he will not benefit from therapy and, in fact, therapy sessions may be counter-productive in this situation. This needs to be carefully explained to the parents, as often they think that progress will be quicker and more effective if the child has more frequent, and longer, therapy sessions.

We have also found that baths, massage, and aromatherapy help relax the child in the evening. The use of aromatherapy oils is discussed with the medical staff for each individual child to ensure that there are no specific medical contraindications (e.g. camphor, hyssop, sage, and rosemary should not be used if the child has experienced, or is likely to experience, epileptic seizures).

Eating and drinking

- What was their diet like, and what are (or were) their favourite (and least favourite) food and drink?
- How are their nutritional needs being met at the moment? (Initially many children with moderate to severe brain injuries are fed via a nasogastric tube).

The child may have difficulty swallowing (dysphagia) which may be related to neurological damage following the brain injury or due to local problems with the mouth, jaw, tongue, or teeth. Feeding (sucking, chewing and swallowing) is assessed as soon as possible after transfer to the neurology ward by the speech therapist with the aid of videofluroscopy, a radiological test which is performed as the child sucks, chews, and swallows. Until they are able to effectively and, more importantly, safely coordinate their swallowing reflex, the child will continue to be fed via a nasogastric tube. Although this may cause the child (and his family) considerable frustration, it is vital to prevent the risk of aspiration of food and liquid into the lungs. If the child has difficulty swallowing his saliva and other secretions then hyoscine is used to reduce these secretions particularly in the initial stages. There are implications for mouth care for the child receiving naso-gastric feeds and mouthwash should be included in oral hygiene care; the nurse must also be aware of the possibility of the child developing oral thrush.

Early and close liaison with the dietitian or nutritionalist will ensure that the appropriate feeding regime is established and that the child is receiving adequate and appropriate nutrition. It is equally important that the child is not over as well as under fed and therefore the child's weight should be monitored weekly.

Many parents wish to learn the procedures involved in nasogastric feeding and a training programme has been established for teaching parents this skill, along with a simple instruction booklet. Not suprisingly, many parents are a little reluctant (usually through fear) to learn this technique, and for children who may require long-term nasogastric feeding this will need to be addressed – preferably as early as possible.

Brain-injured children often experience problems with gastro-oesophageal reflux, which may require specific drug treatment (including Gaviscon and cisapride), as well as dietary manipulation. Should the child need long-term nasogastric feeding then a gastrostomy tube is often preferred to a nasogastric tube. An additional surgical technique which is sometimes required is a fundoplication if gastro-oesophageal reflux is an additional and major problem. A number of children with severe brain injuries frequently develop additional non-specific, but clearly painful or uncomfortable, gastrointestinal symptoms (including flatus, colic, and diarrhoea), some of which have an obvious cause (e.g. the type of diet they are receiving or an episode of gastroenteritis), whilst others have no clear aetiology. In these situations advice is usually sought from the hospital's 'feeding-clinic' team.

As the child's swallowing reflex returns and he is able to protect his airway then a diet is introduced, often beginning with solids as these are easier to control than fluids. It is usually necessary to supplement the oral intake with nasogastric feeds until he has have achieved his required calorie intake. The child will also require additional fluids to provide his necessary fluid requirements. Careful monitoring of the fluid balance is particularly important if the child has definite or suspected diabetes insipidus.

Elimination

- Was the child continent (including toilet-trained) prior to the brain injury, and what was his usual bowel pattern?
- Are there any current problems? (As with any relatively or completely immobile patient, constipation can frequently pose a significant problem and the child may require one or more laxatives. In the majority of patients these can usually be discontinued once mobility has returned and the child is eating a more normal diet. Conversely, diarrhoea may be more of a problem, particularly if the child is fed exclusively nasogastrically or in the first few days and weeks following the insertion of a feeding gastrostomy.)
- Did the child have any previous problems with bladder control or urine infections?
- Is the child currently incontinent and how is this being addressed; is the child catheterized or, as is more commonly the case on transfer, is he wearing nappies or a pad? (This is an area that needs to be addressed sensitively in the older child with the objective being, wherever possible, to maintain privacy and dignity. Toileting often has to be re-established and it is important to start a regular toileting routine as early as possible, depending upon the child's level of awareness and any relevant physical injuries.)

If the child is passing excessive amounts of urine (polyuria), with or without drinking excessively (polydipsia), then diabetes insipidus should be suspected. This is a recognized complication of a brain injury (usually a traumatic head injury, but also following encephalitis and some brain tumours) and is due to a failure of secretion of the antidiuretic hormone (also called vasopressin or DDAVP) from the posterior pituitary gland. It can be confirmed or excluded by measuring the concentration (osmolality) of the blood and urine. Treatment includes a careful fluid balance and replacing the hormone either by tablet or nasal drops/spray. Diabetes insipidus complicating a traumatic or non-traumatic brain injury may be temporary or permanent.

Personal hygiene and dress

- Does the child normally have a bath or shower and at what time of day?
- Does he need any special bath additives, e.g. oilatum for eczema?
- How will hygiene needs be met at this time – is a bath seat required to support the child in the bath, is a mobile hoist required for the older child and does he need a shower chair or trolley? (These issues are addressed jointly by the nursing staff, physiotherapist, and occupational therapist.)

Soon after transfer to the neurology ward, parents are asked to bring in the child's usual clothes rather than the child wearing nightclothes through the day. Good shoes or trainers are needed for when they stand independently or in a frame.

A major component of the rehabilitation process is to promote independence and washing and dressing is one of the key areas. The child is taught strategies to cope with any disabilities; e.g. if they have a left-sided weakness then they are taught to put their left arm in their sleeves before their right. Occupational therapists ensure an effective, and importantly, a consistent dressing strategy amongst everyone who is involved in the day to day care and management of the child.

Skin integrity

- Are there any problems with the child's skin integrity?

When the child is immobile, frequent changes in position are necessary for his comfort but also to relieve pressure. Pressure relieving aids, particularly mattresses and special beds (e.g. Clinitron® and occasionally waterbeds), may be extremely useful in the early stages of rehabilitation.

If the child has sustained a traumatic brain injury, there may be additional injuries including cuts, lacerations, and compound fractures. These will need to be treated appropriately and if dressings are required, it may necessitate deferring hydrotherapy until the injuries have healed.

Pressure areas will obviously need to be observed carefully whenever splints or orthoses have been used to treat contractures and fractures, and also on the occipital area of the scalp where alopecia (hair loss) may have developed as a result of friction from tapes which may have been used to secure the endotracheal tube in place if the child had required ventilatory support.

Contractures

If the child has sustained a severe brain injury (irrespective of whether traumatic or atraumatic), contractures may develop early and may be severe. As well as splints and orthoses (which may need to be altered or modified throughout the rehabilitation programme), pharmacotherapy (i.e. drug therapy) may also be required. This may include anti-spasticity drugs (e.g. baclofen, dantrolene, or a benzodiazepine used singly or in combination) and more locally-acting drugs such as botulinum toxin which can be injected into the most severely contracted (and therefore painful) muscles. (The use of botulinum toxin in this situation is still largely investigational and should only be carried out by doctors who are experienced in this technique.) In most children the use of any of these drugs is for a limited period. However, other children with more severe brain injuries may require long-term treatment and even, ultimately, surgery to more effectively treat particularly marked and painful and functionally disabling contractures.

Controlling body temperature

- Is the child's temperature within normal limits?
- What are the usual antipyretic measures taken by the parents when the child is pyrexial?
- Does the child have a tendency (at home) to be warm or cold at night? (It is usually appropriate to bring in his favourite bedclothes, including a duvet or duvet covers.)

An abnormally high (or low) temperature which persists in the first few days or weeks following the injury may be due to an underlying focus of infection (particularly chest or urine) or simply reflect an instability of the centres within the brain (principally the hypothalamus) which are responsible for controlling the body temperature. Marked swings (up or down) of the temperature are usually more suggestive of a 'central control' problem, whilst a persistently high temperature is more commonly associated with an underlying infection, which should be sought. The possibility of meningitis or a cerebral abscess must also be considered, particularly if the child had experienced a traumatic brain injury complicated by a depressed or basal skull fracture or requiring neurosurgical intervention. Additional causes in children with non- or atraumatic injuries (e.g: due to meningitis or encephalitis) could include a recurrence or relapse of these infections due to partial or inadequate treatment; this is a well-recognized complication of herpes simplex encephalitis.

Mobilizing

- Was the child walking/crawling prior to the injury, and were there any pre-existing problems with his balance or gait?
- Does the child have any additional injury that could influence mobilisation (e.g. fractures or severe abrasions and lacerations)?

Close liaison with the physiotherapists is clearly necessary at the beginning of, and throughout, the rehabilitation programme to determine the rate of mobilization and pattern of exercises allowed, as well as deciding which splints should be used and when.

Seating is an important issue because the child may have difficulty sitting unsupported for a number of reasons, including spasticity. The physiotherapist and occupational therapist will advise on the most appropriate seating and standing frames, as well as the most suitable wheelchairs and buggies. It is clearly impossible to have every possible chair that may be needed, but the rehabilitation unit has attempted to establish a supply of chairs which may be easily adapted to satisfy the individual child's requirements. As these requirements can change rapidly (weekly or even daily) it is not advisable to purchase individual chairs until each child's long-term needs become much clearer. If at that point, specialized seating is still required, the child will be referred to the relevant community seating and wheelchair clinic.

Communicating

Did the child have any pre-existing hearing or speech/language difficulties? What is the child's dominant language (e.g. English or Welsh, Urdu or Cantonese, etc.)?

Communication problems are relatively common and may be either receptive (where the child has difficulty understanding speech) or expressive (where the child has difficulty in speaking and in expressing himself), or both. The terms 'aphasia' and 'dysphasia' are used to indicate a total lack of (aphasia), or difficulty with (dysphasia), the comprehension or production of communication. Fortunately, the vast majority of communication difficulties are temporary and permanent difficulties are usually expressive rather than receptive in nature, although both may obviously occur simultaneously. The speech and language therapist is involved as early as necessary, and dependent on the child's needs, to ensure that the appropriate communication aids are used as well as liaising with the nursing, playstaff, and other therapists regarding coping strategies on a day-to-day basis.

Parents, family, and friends are encouraged to talk to the child about the everyday events, recount past events, and to talk about friends, as well as about what is happening now, including the day and date. This helps to establish if the child has problems with his short-or long-term memory. The child's favourite story or music tapes and books are also brought in; these are often most useful during the early stages of the rehabilitation programme

There will always be a number of children who will have missed their birthday or Christmas following their brain injury due to their injuries and lack of awareness, and when they have become more aware they are convinced that these events have not yet occurred. Once they discover that they have missed them they feel cheated, and on many occasions these special events will be celebrated a 'second' time for the child.

Expressing sexuality

Again this relates to age, and older children in particular may have boyfriends or girlfriends and will want to spend time on their own with each other. Wherever possible, this should be respected and they should be given privacy, including the opportunity of being on their own if they so wish. It is clearly important that children should be dressed appropriately for their age – and again, it is encouraged that the child's own clothes are worn throughout their hospital admission.

In the acute phase of recovery the child may be very disinhibited, both verbally and even physically. Clearly this should be explained to parents, often forewarning them that this behaviour is neither unexpected nor uncommon, but usually only for a limited period. Many parents find this very difficult to understand or accept and become understandably distressed; psychological support (for the family – and occasionally for the ward staff!) and intervention is sought if this phase of the child's recovery persists.

Spiritual needs

Some families find that their religion provides them with strength and support and obviously this should be encouraged and facilitated. Others do not, and again this must be understood and respected.

Thinking and feeling

It is very helpful to try and gain some degree of insight into the child's personality prior to the injury; were they quiet or extrovert; what were the types of issues that would worry him (and how were these usually addressed); and, conversely, what were the activities that he found supportive and comforting? Many families have videos of their child prior to the injury, and these can sometimes provide a valuable insight for the nurse regarding the child's personality and 'character' prior to the injury.

- Did the child have negative feelings towards professionals, such as doctors or nurses, or fears of hospitals or tests which may have followed a previously unhappy or distressing experience in hospital?
- What is his feeling or concept about body image, and in particular, his reaction to any disfigurement or disability, including the weakness or even loss of a limb which may have occurred as a complication of his brain injury (e.g. after a road traffic accident, or during an illness such as meningococcal septicaemia)? (Both the child and the family may need considerable support in coming to terms with a disability, particularly if there has been a loss of a whole, or part of, a limb.)

Following a brain injury, children may demonstrate a number of changes in their behaviour and personality. The parents may become overprotective and hence overly restrictive or they may become more indulgent with the child. This can frequently confuse the child as the normal parental discipline and control has changed, which may further complicate the child – parent relationship and understanding; this is discussed in more detail later in the book.

Playing

- What type of play did the child enjoy; was he sporty or did he enjoy quiet games?
- What are his favourite toys?
- Did he prefer to play with other children or to play on his own?

Finding out about favourite radio and television programmes and specific heroes (e.g: sporting, TV, or musical) enables the nurse (and other members of the team) to talk to the child about familiar things, so helping to develop and establish a good rapport.

For most children, play is extremely important and is frequently used as a measure or technique to facilitate the introduction of the child (as well as the family) to the rehabilitation programme and to members of the rehabilitation team. This requires close liaison between the play therapists and the nurses/ therapists. This is now discussed in more detail.

Play-intervention programmes

Liaison with the therapists provides the play specialist with information which is integral to the application of play intervention programmes. These programmes initially consist of a series of activities to stimulate the child if there are specific areas of concern. For example, in the early stages of rehabilitation caring for a child who does not appear to respond physically or intellectually, the most appropriate programme for stimulation may consist of very basic or primitive activities to stimulate the senses of touch, smell, taste, vision, and hearing. Sensory play helps refresh senses which may have been dulled or temporarily impaired through trauma, and incorporate the use of:

- tactile materials of different textures to stimulate touch and feel
- various food tastes
- different smells
- visual stimulation which may include the use of the multi-sensory (Snooezlen®) room to 'visually excite' and to encourage the child to fix, focus, and track or follow visual stimuli.

Additional early treatment may include the use of aromatherapy massage to aid the child who may be experiencing periods of restlessness and distress. It can be particularly soothing when used with Snooezlen® music to promote relaxation, and if applied each evening, it frequently assists in the establishment of a regular and sustained sleep pattern.

As the rehabilitation process progresses, the play programme is adjusted to meet the individual child's needs. A child with limited gross movements or a hemiplegia may begin with simple activities of pushing a beach ball on a table or pushing a balloon, rolling play dough or other malleable materials, progressing to more strenuous activities such as basketball which helps to stimulate and strengthen large arm movements. The child may then progress to specific activities aimed at redeveloping fine manipulation skills, including drawing, sewing, threading and the use of games (e.g: jigsaws and other puzzles) which contain small pieces and which require pincer grip and good finger control for their completion.

Short-term memory, concentration, and cognitive/intellectual skills are stimulated and, as is often necessary, redeveloped using a wide range of activities which may be oral, written, or computer-based. The computer activities (often in the form of games) are particularly popular with the older child or teenager who do not regard the games as promoting memory skills and hand – eye coordination but as an interesting, familiar and favourite occupation.

The play specialist will frequently accompany the child to their different therapy sessions to liaise with the therapists in considering any additional and therapy-directed activities that can be incorporated into the ward-based play programme.

The importance of play

Play may be used simply to ease communication with children. Play enables them to become more relaxed and spontaneous when both the child and the adult are concentrating on a third object. This may be in the form of an interest or hobby, a toy or a game that the child is interested in, or simply a shared outing providing neutral ground to gain the child's attention and promote confidence between the child and staff.

Children undergoing rehabilitation who have shown regression as a result of their brain injury will usually require structured play at a younger level than their chronological age. Clearly, the level of play will change and adapt to reflect the child's progress.

A common view of childrens' play is that it is somehow trivial and unimportant; however, all children play and it is through the important medium of play that they develop and mature physically, emotionally, and even intellectually. Research has shown a clear and direct link between hospital play and an increase in the speed of recovery (Jolly 1975; Plank 1964) through a reduction in anxiety experienced by the child (Billington 1972; Garot 1986). Play specialists do far more than occupy children; they can reduce uncertainty and distress by providing play that is familiar and a welcome relief after all the strange and confusing sights, sounds, and bodily discomfort which they may experience in hospital.

Play can also be beneficial to siblings who may experience a loss of attention and containment because of the parents' understandable focus and emphasis on the ill child, and who may, as a result, spend long periods of time on the hospital ward.

Play preparation

The child may have to undergo further tests and investigations and again it is often the play specialists who will reduce the child's anxiety by preparing the child with simple explanations through play, preparation toys, slides or photographs, and, when necessary, sound effects. For example, for those children who need a magnetic resonance imaging (MRI) brain scan, a tape of the noise made by the scanner will be played to the child while they play with a model of the scanner (including a Barbie doll) to facilitate the child's cooperation with the test. When this is successful the child will usually lie quietly, without moving, therefore obviating the need for sedation or a general anaesthetic. Preparation of the child facing further investigations can also prevent misunderstanding and reduce unnecessary anxiety. Finally, such preparation again redresses the balance of power in favour of the child. Focused play in preparation helps the child assimilate information and gain mastery.

Social needs (socialisation)

- What is the family structure?
- Who are the most important people in the child's life? (Understandably, and not infrequently, this includes a grandparent or an aunt/uncle.)

- What are the names and ages of any siblings; how can they be involved; and how are they coping with the situation?
- Does the child have any pets? (The parents may like to bring in photographs and, depending on the pet, visits to the ward can sometimes be arranged.)
- What school or nursery does the child attend? (Teachers from the hospital school will always liaise with the child's school to find out about his previous abilities (academic and physical) and any problems, including whether the child had any special educational needs. Many children who have suffered traumatic brain injury (i.e: a head injury) will be found to have had pre-existing learning or behavioural difficulties before the injury. (A significant number will be said to have been easily distractable and unable to concentrate for any length of time.)
- Did they socialize/mix well at school? (Friends and classmates should be encouraged to visit, but if the child has any significant problems, friends will need to be told before they visit about his condition and the fact that he may or may not be aware of their presence or understand their reactions. Although younger children usually find these situations easier to accept, older children can sometimes be less tolerant and therefore less sensitive, because of their own preconceptions.)
- Have other health care professionals been involved previously with the family and child (for any reason), such as a district nurse, health visitor, or social worker? (A social worker is a key member of our team and routinely offers early support and advice to the family if their child has suffered a brain injury; this will clearly be done in conjunction with any other social worker who already knows the family.)

During the child's rehabilitation it is often recognized that the child may become bored and even frustrated; this is occasionally expressed as challenging or 'difficult' behaviour or even as 'withdrawal'. At such times, an outing appropriate to the child's condition and level of comprehension may overcome this particular problem. Visits to the park for younger children, or to the circus, pantomime, or cinema provide an enjoyable activity and although these represent a break from the routine of hospital rehabilitation they are still important in the overall programme. Trips to the cinema, theatre, tenpin bowling, and their favourite restaurants (usually of the fast food variety!) help the adolescent to regain social skills, including mixing and (often) relearning acceptable public behaviour. Initially these outings may be traumatic because the child may be a little fearful and apprehensive of venturing outside the hospital environment; they may show a loss of confidence, and in some cases difficulty in understanding and accepting impaired physical skills, with consequent frustration, anger, and withdrawal.

Planning activities to accentuate the positive rather than the negative aspects of his abilities may help the child come to terms with any reduced skills, thus building his confidence and providing positive feedback. It has been found that if a child can become convinced that his disability is only relative, half of the therapeutic battle is won (Hallers 1970). However, this may be particularly difficult for adolescents who are usually fully aware of their reduced skills and abilities and are often acutely (and over-) sensitive to the public's response to these disabilities.

The family may also experience difficulty in coping with their child's difficulties and disabilities and also in accepting the attitude of both friends and strangers. The team recognize that this is a common problem and to help overcome this a series of outings or visits are arranged for both the child and the family, but also including the primary nurse and play specialist to support the family through this difficult period of adjustment. The family and child may need to learn a series of coping strategies which can be achieved by observing how staff themselves cope with people who may appear curious and insensitive about the child's problems. A disability that is seen within the context of the hospital environment often seems far more acceptable than when it is encountered within the normal everyday situation outside this safe environment; this again emphasizes the importance of the various visits and trips to public places using a gradual and 'desensitizing' approach.

Maintaining a safe environment

Many children are agitated or confused in the period following the injury and may require padded cot or bed sides to prevent them injuring themselves. Cot sides and a protective helmet may also be required if the child is experiencing epileptic seizures, particularly if these are frequent or poorly controlled.

- Was the child mischievous prior to the injury and is he likely to do as he is asked or is he likely to show off and dare to do what he has been told not to do? (As mentioned earlier, a significant number of children who have suffered a traumatic brain injury will be found to have had pre-existing learning or behavioural difficulties before the injury. A number will be said to have been clumsy or to have been impulsive. In our own experience of over 110 children with a head injury treated in the rehabilitation programme, approximately 75% were found to have pre-existing learning difficulties, behaviour problems, or both. It is likely that these pre-existing problems could have contributed to the injury in the first place by making them less aware of, or less able to escape from, any potentially dangerous situation or activity.)

Additional problems

It is not possible to discuss these additional problems in full detail – but it is important that those people working with brain-injured children are aware of them (Piek 1995).

Epilepsy

Epilepsy may arise as a complication of any brain injury – whether traumatic (see below) or atraumatic. Encephalitis (Annegers *et al.* 1988) is one of the most common causes of acquired, non-traumatic epilepsy; other causes include meningitis (Annegers et al. 1988; Rosman *et al.* 1985), as a result of a hypoxic – ischaemic insult to the brain (e.g. following a cardiac arrest or a near drowning accident) or due to a biochemical disturbance (e.g. hypogly-caemia – a low blood sugar). Occasionally, the seizures will cease as soon as the insult has resolved, as in the case of most biochemical or metabolic disturbances. However, epileptic seizures that follow encephalitis or menin-gitis may recur (even weeks or months after the insult has occurred) and may then need to be treated with anti-epileptic drugs.

Seizures that follow a traumatic brain injury (i.e. a head injury) - called post-traumatic epilepsy – are more common and therefore deserve a specific comment (Annegers et al., 1980; Dugan and Howell 1994; Jennett 1973; Kieslich and Jacobi 1995; Temkin *et al* 1995).

The majority of children (and adults) who have a head injury do not experience a seizure (also called a convulsion or fit). There is surprisingly little information on the incidence of epilepsy arising as a consequence of head injuries, and what does exist is over 20 years old (Jennett 1973); however, it is based on a large number of subjects – 1000 consecutive and unselected children. The overall risk of epilepsy following a head injury is approxi-mately 5%; it is slightly higher (between 7 and 9%) in children less than 5 years of age. This should be compared with the incidence of epilepsy in children who have not experienced a head injury, which is 0.7 – 0.8%.

Post-traumatic seizures can be classified into three types:

(1) immediate – seizures occurring within seconds or minutes of the injury;
(2) early – seizures occurring within the first week of the injury;
(3) late – seizures occurring months to years following the injury.

The incidence of immediate or early seizures varies between 5% and 20%, depending on the severity of the injury. Immediate and early seizures occur with about equal frequency in the first hour after injury, in the rest of the first day, and in the remainder of the first week. Importantly, early seizures are one of the major risk factors predisposing to the development of later seizures (called 'late epilepsy'). There are a number of additional factors which are associated with an increased risk of late epilepsy:

● immediate/early seizures
● depressed skull fracture (the edge of the fracture is forced down into the brain)

- intracranial haemorrhage/haematoma
- prolonged (i.e. > 24 hours) post-traumatic amnesia (PTA)
- focal cerebral damage
- severe diffuse cerebral damage
- genetic predisposition towards epilepsy.

As expected, the greater number of factors, the greater is the chance of developing late epilepsy. Early post-traumatic seizures are correlated with a 25–40% risk of late seizures (late epilepsy). This rate increases to almost 50% if there has been an intracranial haemorrhage and up to 60% if most of the above factors have occurred. Prolonged post-traumatic amnesia and a genetic predisposition to epilepsy (as manifest by a family history of epilepsy) do not, *in isolation*, increase the risk of late epilepsy in the absence of all the other risk factors. It is important to realize that all of the above risk factors are related to the primary brain injury. If there is any secondary brain damage, this will further increase the risk of both early and late seizures.

Investigations, including electroencephalography (EEG) and brain imaging (computerized tomography [CT]) are not entirely reliable predictors of late epilepsy. It is possible that in the future, more sophisticated methods of imaging the brain, such as diffusion-weighted magnetic resonance imaging (MRI) or single photon emission computerized tomography (SPECT) or positron emission tomography (PET) may prove to be more accurate (and reliable) methods of predicting which children will be more likely to develop late epilepsy.

Approximately 20% of children with late seizures will have their initial seizure in the first month after the injury whilst 50–60% of late seizures will develop within the first year; the majority of these children will have experienced one or more early seizures. Approximately 20% of children will still develop late epilepsy as long as 4 years after the injury, and the figure will have fallen to 10% or less by 6 years or longer.

The types of seizures that children experience may be complex partial (also called focal, affecting one part of the brain only, and therefore only one part/half of the body), primary generalized (affecting both halves of the brain, and therefore the whole body, simultaneously) and secondary generalized (when the seizure may start as a partial seizure but then 'spreads' to the rest of the brain, resulting in a secondary generalized tonic-clonic ['grand mal'] convulsion). The majority of early seizures are partial seizures, and over half of all late seizures are generalized (more commonly secondary rather than primary generalized), seizures. Partial seizures may take the form of prolonged absences or altered, confused behaviour with semi-purposeful actions. They may sometimes be difficult to diagnose, particularly if the child already has learning difficulties or an abnormal behaviour profile which might have been present before the head injury, or have arisen as a direct consequence of the injury. It is therefore important to be as certain as possible before a diagnosis of epilepsy is made in this population. Status epilepticus (which means a prolonged tonic-clonic convulsion lasting more than 30 minutes) is more likely to occur in the first few days after the injury and is seen more often in children than in adults, particularly if under 2 years of age.

In the past, there has been much debate regarding the use of anti-epileptic drugs (AEDs) to prevent the development of late epilepsy. Current evidence suggests that the use of AEDs does not reduce the risk – and incidence – of late epilepsy (Young *et al.* 1983); in fact, in one adult study of over 400 patients, over 27% of patients treated with an AED had developed late epilepsy at 2 years following the head injury, in contrast to only 21% of patients who had not received an AED. However, the same study provided evidence that giving an anti-epileptic drug just for the first week after the head injury could reduce the risk of further seizures occurring in that week (Temkin *et al.* 1990). It is our current practice to prescribe phenytoin (initially intravenously) if the child has had two or more seizures in the first few days following the head injury and to discontinue the drug after 6 or 8 weeks if the child has remained seizure-free.

It is clearly important to discuss this issue with parents and to advise them on the relative risks of their child developing epilepsy, how the seizures may present (i.e: what the seizures could look like if and when they occur), and what first aid measures they should take, if their child has a seizure. Should late post-traumatic epilepsy develop, the anti-epileptic drug of choice will depend on the type of seizure and EEG findings, but should *not* include phenytoin, pheno-barbitone, or the benzodiazepines as the drugs of first choice.

Fractures

Fractured limbs are not uncommon additional injuries, particularly in association with other severe injuries, usually resulting from road traffic accidents or falls from heights. Such fractures may interfere with the rehabilitation programme for a number of reasons, including pain and discomfort, immobilization (often with traction), and delay in functional recovery, particularly if there is neurological dysfunction of the non-fractured limb(s).

Skull fractures rarely cause any problem, assuming that any depressed fracture has been appropriately cleaned and elevated. However, there may be a residual defect in the skull, either because of a severe and compound or comminuted skull fracture or because of an emergency craniotomy and decompression of an acutely swollen brain. Although it is likely that this defect will be subsequently repaired (using either the patient's own bone or a titanium plate), this may not be for some weeks or even months. During this time the child's parents may be understandably concerned that the brain underlying the skull fracture and defect is relatively unprotected; parents can,

and should be reassured that in the vast majority of situations this
constitute any signficiant risk or problem, although certain contact s....
rugby and boxing) should be avoided!

Spinal injuries *(particularly of the cervical spine)*

These must *always* be considered in any child who has suffered a head injury
and be excluded (or confirmed) by appropriate radiological investigation.
Occasionally, subluxation or even dislocation of the cervical spine may be
missed (with potentially tragic consequences) due to the focus of medical/
surgical attention on the head injury.

Infections

This includes methicillin-resistant *Staphylococcus aureus* – or MRSA – a type of
bacterial infection which is becoming increasingly common in hospital and is
difficult to treat because it is resistant to most, if not all, antibiotics. The child
usually needs to be nursed in a cubicle away from other children and this can
delay many components of the rehabilitation programme – particularly hydrotherapy – but also other therapies as well as attendance at the hospital school.

THE CARE PLAN

Following the initial assessment, the primary nurse and parents negotiate an
agreed plan of care for the child according to the needs that have been identified.
It is important to establish how involved in the child's care the family wish to be at
the beginning and throughout the rehabilitation programme. The level of
involvement will change, often on a daily or weekly basis, as families gain in
confidence and want to take on more aspects of the child's care. It is important to
prevent nurses taking over all the child's care and also to ensure that the nurse
does not put undue pressure on the family to undertake more care than they feel
that they can manage. Importantly, parental involvement in the child's care
should not be regarded as being a substitute for nurses, or for reducing the need
for appropriate staffing levels. Just because a parent has developed the necessary
skills to give their child a nasogastric feed does not mean that they are expected to
undertake that aspect of care all the time. There are some aspects of care that the
older child would not feel comfortable for their parents to do and the nurse and
parents need to be aware of this and together identify areas where this may apply.
    When considering their approach to the child and parents, all members of
the team need to take into account a number of factors, including the
circumstances of the injury, level of consciousness, awareness of the environment, fear, irritation and frustration experienced by the child, family circumstances, social factors, and level of family participation in the rehabilitation

because all of these factors may affect the child's response. As with any care plan, discharge planning will start on the child's admission to the unit.

HEAD-INJURY PROGRESS CHART

The play specialist will assess if it is appropriate to implement a head injury progress chart (Figs 4.1 and 4.2), encompassing all areas of the rehabilitation

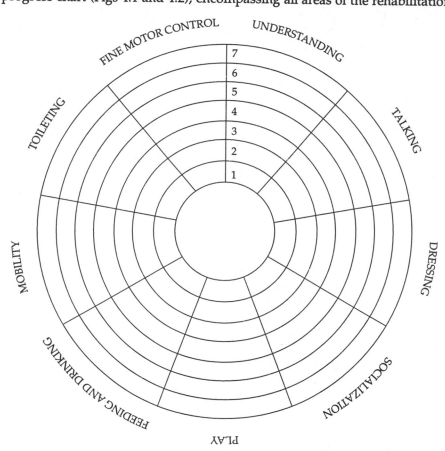

Fig. 4.1 Head (brain) injury progress chart. The child's different levels of ability in the nine categories are graded from 1 to 7, with 1 the lowest, and 7 the highest level of ability (see Box 4.1). As the child's recovery progresses, the chart is completed appropriately – usually by the child's parents or by the nursing staff or play therapists. It must be emphasised that this is a non-standard method of monitoring the child's recovery and is easily presented in a visual format, predominantly (but not exclusively) for the benefit of the family. (Adapted with modifications from the 'Keele Pre-School Assessment Guide'; Tyler, S. (1980). Keele Pre-School Assessment Guide. NFER-Nelson, Windsor).

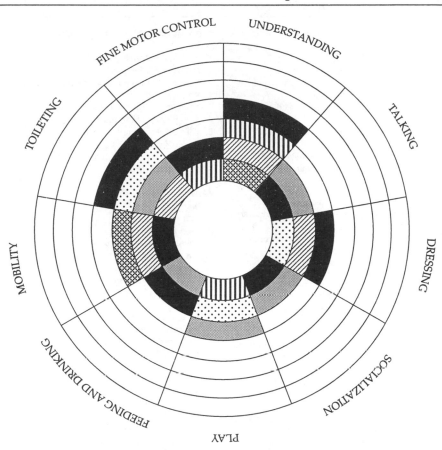

Fig. 4.2 Example of how the head (brain) injury progress chart is completed for one particular child. In practice, the different 'segments' would be coloured, and not shaded.

process. The chart was drawn together by the play specialists, in conjunction with team-members, to reflect a step-by-step approach to the skills which the team members consider appropriate in assessing the child's rehabilitation progress. The chart is simple to use by parents who colour-code and date the child's progress in each area. Parental contribution to the chart allows them to actively participate in their child's rehabilitation and to monitor his progress, thereby enabling them to reflect on the rehabilitation process; thus, if and when the recovery process appears slow and laborious, the chart will be able to demonstrate the extent of progress that their child has made.

Box 4.1 Different levels of ability in the head (brain) injury progress chart

Understanding
1. No apparent understanding
2. Listens to familiar sounds and voices
3. Responds to 'tone of voice'
4. Can identify familiar people and objects on request
5. Understands simple requests with situational cues
6. Understands simple requests without cues
7. Understands general conversation

Talking
1. No apparent communication
2. Cries and moans when uncomfortable/ upset
3. Uses sounds, facial expression, body language to communicate
4. Uses gestures, signs, pictures to communicate
5. Uses single words
6. Uses simple sentences
7. Joins in general conversation

Dressing
1. Helps with dressing by holding out arm for sleeve and foot for shoe
2. Helps move constructively with dressing
3. Takes off shoes, socks, hat – seldom able to replace
4. Puts on hat and gloves
5. Takes part more actively with dressing but still needs help with fastenings
6. Can dress and undress except for laces, ties, and back buttons
7. Undresses and dresses alone

Socialization
1. Shows no awareness
2. Shows awareness of people/events
3. Responds to familiar people
4. Initiates interactions
5. Responds to new people
6. Initiates interaction with new people
7. Joins in small group activities

Play
1. Observes play
2. Solitary play
3. Parallel play
4. Interactive play
5. Group play
6. Initiates play
7. Independent play

Feeding and Drinking
1. Nasogastric feeds only
2. Nasogastric feeds with some semi-solids from spoon
3. Thickened drinks from open cup
4. Finely chopped foods from fork or spoon
5. Thin drinks from open cup
6. Finger foods
7. Eats usual range of foods using appropriate utensils

Mobility
1. Immobile
2. Sits with support
3. Stands with support
4. Takes steps with support
5. Stands alone
6. Walks alone
7. Walks up and down stairs.

Toileting
1. Wears protection
2. Indicates when wet or dry
3. Indicates the need for the toilet
4. Asks for the toilet
5. Bladder control
6. Toilet-trained with infrequent accidents/ night time
7. Goes to toilet alone

Fine motor control
1. Palmar grasp and transfer, manipulates smalls toys
2. Grasps between finger and thumb scissor fashion
3. Pincer grasp, points with index finger
4. Manipulates cubes, builds tower of two
5. Holds pencil mid-shaft with palmar or tripod grasp, builds tower of three cubes
6. Picks up small objects quickly and neatly. Removes paper from sweet. Builds tower of six to seven cubes
7. Builds nine-cube tower, threads beads, six piece circle, imitates cross

THE MEDIA

Frequently, when a child has sustained a brain injury and particularly if there has been some drama attached to it (e.g: a hit and run road-traffic accident, or as the result of a rare or puzzling serious illness), the media often look for a story. No information is given to the media without the permission of the parents. When the child is still in the intensive-care unit, information is usually provided with the use of standard and 'acceptable' terms, including critical, stable, comfortable, etc.

Once transferred to the ward for rehabilitation the media usually want pictures of the child with or without the parents and even with some of the rehabilitation team. Occasionally, some families do actively encourage media interest, others have been happy to speak to the media when approached, whilst others do not want any media involvement at all. The team's primary responsibility is to the child first and the family second. Although the family will be supported in whichever approach to the media they choose to take, if the child is upset or distressed by the attention then media interest will be discouraged and the parents and family will be advised to do the same, although obviously they can do as they wish outside the hospital.

LITIGATION

The nature of some children's injuries may mean that the family are involved in litigation procedures. The team do not become directly involved in these procedures on a day to day basis because the rehabilitation of the child is their foremost concern; however, statements may have to be given to the police (particularly if the child has suffered a non-accidental head injury) and legal reports may occasionally be required, again usually if the child has sustained a head injury as a result of a road-traffic accident.

Parents may, understandably, show a mistrust of health care professionals if the brain injury has been as a result of negligent practice. The team will obviously support families but without showing bias or favour, and will endeavour to gain their trust and respect whilst understanding the bitterness and anger they sometimes feel.

PARENT SUPPORT GROUPS

Parents who have previously been through the experience of having a brain-injured child admitted to the HIRT programme (months or even years earlier), will often readily come into the ward and speak to newly 'bereaved' parents at the beginning of, and throughout, the rehabilitation programme. They are able to empathize with the family and share some of their feelings of grief, anxiety, and fears. Parents frequently benefit from meeting other families who have faced and dealt with similar problems and appreciate the opportunity to talk through some of their emotions. It is very useful to meet and talk to others who have 'been there' and have 'come through' the difficulties that they are currently experiencing.

A more formal parent support group has been established by the HIRT social worker and head injury 'link' school teacher, which is well-attended and has been of tremendous benefit to many families. The group meet either within the hospital (in the parent accommodation block rather than the ward) or in someone's home – or even (rarely) in a pub. Parents are also informed of the national head injury groups, specifically the Children's Head Injury Trust (CHIT) and Headway, if they would like to talk to other families outside Liverpool or obtain further written information and advice. The HIRT also tries to develop close links with these organizations.

DISCHARGE PLANNING

As with any patient, it is important to consider discharge plans and requirements early rather than later. Clearly, there will be limitations to how detailed these plans can be, particularly in the early stages of the rehabilitation programme, because it will not be known (or necessarily predicted) at what point the child's recovery will plateau and what specific aids or adaptations to the home will be required on discharge. However, for a number of children it will be easier to predict their needs on discharge and as meeting these needs may take some time, the sooner they are discussed and planned, the better.

Discharging the child home is frequently a difficult and traumatic time – both physically and emotionally. Initially, a home visit is arranged for a few hours, then an overnight stay, and, depending on the severity of the child's brain injury, degree of recovery, and family circumstances this is gradually extended to weekend leave. Occasionally, the child may remain as an in-patient within the rehabilitation programme on a Monday to Thursday or Friday basis, returning home for weekends; this is frequently the arrangement for children referred to the HIRT from outside Liverpool (e.g: from Cumbria, Shropshire, and Herefordshire). Eventually, when all involved with the child's rehabilitation (particularly the parents) are happy, the child is discharged from the in-patient phase of the programme, although he may continue to attend the hospital as a day-patient to receive continuing therapy and schooling; this day-patient phase may last days, weeks, or months, depending on the severity of the child's injury, his response to therapy and the family's usual place of residence.

It is common practice to provide some short-term loan of nursing equipment, including commodes and wheelchairs, to facilitate these early – and important – home visits and periods of weekend leave.

It is obviously important to ensure that the community and primary health-care teams are kept informed of the child's progress, particularly if it is likely that the child will be an in-patient (or day-patient, or both) for a considerable time or will have significant physical and educational needs at the time of discharge from the hospital ward. This will include notifying and updating the general practitioner, community paediatrician, community paediatric/district nurses, community therapists, health visitors, and school nurses. This enables everyone to be made aware of not only the child's progress but also the possible implications for siblings and the entire family, who may themselves require continuing support and advice.

For children whose home is outside Liverpool and whose brain injury has been serious (with almost certain severe neurological sequelae), the health care professionals from their own community will be invited to visit the ward and attend the early-discharge planning meetings organized by the HIRT at Alder Hey. Many have expressed how useful this has been in facilitating discharge plans and ensuring a smooth hand-over from hospital to community care and continuing rehabilitation, including identifying the most appropriate school placement.

For children who have been left with severe neurological deficits, consideration is given to providing future respite care – either within the hospital (Alder Hey has a separate short-term residential unit for children with severe learning [and other] disabilities), with a foster family, or with social services. There is clear evidence of the stress that caring for children with severe brain damage imposes on the family. Nevertheless, families normally wish to continue to provide long-term care, but assistance in the form of short-term relief and support may obviate the need for long-term residential care (which may be unavailable or too expensive) and prevent unacceptable and intolerable stress on the family (Oddy *et al.* 1989).

Finally, wherever possible we try and arrange that the discharge from the hospital ward to home is never on a Thursday or Friday, in case there are unforeseen medical or nursing problems which may be more difficult to address and resolve over a weekend.

REFERENCES

Appleton, R.E. (1994). Head-Injury rehabilitation for children. *Nursing Times*, **90**, 29–31.

Annegers, J.F., Grabow, J.D., Groover, R.V., Laws Jr., E.R., Elveback, L.R., and Kurland, L.T. (1980). Seizures after head trauma: a population study. *Neurology*, **30**, 683–9.

Annegers, J. F., *et al.* (1988). The risk of unprovoked seizures after encephalitis and meningitis. *Neurology*, **38**, 1407–10.

Billington, G.F. (1972). Play program reduces children's anxiety, speeds recoveries. *Modern Hospital*, **118**, 90–2.

Calef, V. (1959). The child in hospital. Cited in (1975): *The family life of sick children: a study of families coping with chronic childhood disease* (ed. Burton Lindy). Routledge and Keegan, London and Boston.

Davidson, L. (1989). Head-injury, the forgotten injury. *Nursing Times*, **85**, 31–2.

Dittmar, S. (1989). *Rehabilitation nursing: process and application*. CV Mosby, St Louis.

Dugan, E. M. and Howell, J. M. (1994). Post-traumatic seizures. *Emergency Medicine Clinics of North America*, **12**, 1081–87.

Garot, P,A. (1986). Therapeutic play: work of both child and nurse. *Journal of Pediatric Nursing*, **1**, 111–16.

Hallers, J. A. (1970). Sick children and their parents. Cited in (1975): *The family life of sick children: A study of families coping with chronic childhood disease* (ed. Burton Lindy). Routledge and Keegan, London and Boston.

Henderson, V. (1966). *The nature of nursing*. Collier–MacMillan, London.

Jennett, B. (1973). Trauma as a cause of epilepsy in childhood. *Developmental Medicine 'and Child Neurology*, **15**, 56–62.

Jolly, H. (1975). How play in hospital helps a child's recovery. *The Times*, 16th July.

Kieslich, M. and Jacobi, G. (1995). Incidence and risk factors of post-traumatic epilepsy in childhood. *Lancet*, **345**, 187.

Lansdown, R, and Goldman, A. (1988). The psychological care of children with malignant disease. *Journal of Child Psychology and Psychiatry*, **29**, 555–67.

Oddy, M., Bonham, E., McMillan, T., Stroud, A., and Rickard, S. (1989). A comprehensive service for the rehabilitation and long-term care of head injury survivors. *Clinical Rehabilitation*, **3**, 253–9.

Piek, J. (1995). Medical complications in severe head injury. *New Horizons*, **3**, 534–8.

Plank, E.N. (1964). *Working with Children in Hospital*. Tavistock Publication.

Roper, N., Logan, W.W., and Tierney, A.J. (1983). *Using a model for nursing*, (pp. 4–17.). Churchill–Livingstone, London.

Rosman, N.P., Peterson, D. B., Kaye, E. M., and Colton, T. (1985). Seizures in bacterial meningitis : prevalence, patterns, and prognosis. *Pediatric Neurology*, **1**, 278–85.

Temkin, N. R., Dikmen, S. S., Wilensky, A. J., Keihm, J., Chabal, S., and Winn, H. R. (1990). A randomized double-blind study of phenytoin for the prevention of post-traumatic seizures. *New England Journal of Medicine*, **323**, 497–502.

Temkin, N. R., Haglund, M. M., and Winn, H. R. (1995). Causes, prevention and treatment of post-traumatic epilepsy. *New Horizons*, **3**, 518–22.

Winnicott, C. (1968). Communication through play. Cited in: (1992): *The handbook of play therapy* (ed. L McMahon). Routledge, London and New York.

Young, B., Papp, R. P., Norton, J. A., Haack, D., Tibbs, P. A., and Bean, J. R. (1983). Failure of prophylactically administered phenytoin to prevent late post-traumatic seizures. *Journal of Neurosurgery*, **58**, 236–41.

5

Physical (motor and functional) difficulties

Juliet Weston, Eileen Kinley, Bronwen Hughes,
and Sue Fishwick

Introduction

This chapter discusses the gross and fine motor rehabilitation which is aimed at maximizing the child's functional independence. It focuses on the role of physiotherapy and occupational therapy in the early, and intermediate rehabilitation as well as the long – term management. It is important to stress that the identification of any physical difficulties and the subsequent approach and methods employed to treat them are almost invariably multi-disciplinary, involving not only physiotherapy and occupational therapy but also ward nursing staff and play specialists.

EARLY MANAGEMENT

Role of physiotherapy

In the intensive care unit (ICU), the child is usually ventilated and paralysed, and may have respiratory or orthopaedic problems, or both. These factors are important as they may limit early positioning and therapy.

Respiratory problems

These are not uncommon in the brain-injured child who requires ventilatory support, and they have multiple causes:

- associated chest trauma with fractured ribs and a pneumothorax
- aspiration of substances at the time of the injury, leading to upper and subsequently lower respiratory tract infections
- reduction of the cough reflex and motility of the lung cilia (because the child is paralysed), causing an increase in the volume of secretions which may also predispose the child to developing a chest infection
- suctioning (to remove excessive secretions) may cause mucosal damage
- prolonged endotracheal intubation may also cause marked mucosal

inflammation leading to scarring and, ultimately, stenosis (narrowing) of the trachea and larynx.

The development of respiratory problems may significantly increase the extent and duration of any ventilatory support, which may have implications for the child's recovery and initiation of the rehabilitation programme.

It is important that any chest physiotherapy that is required should be carefully timed to minimize the disturbance to the child, with sessions being short and effective and preferably linked into the routine nursing care, e.g. when the child is turned or washed.

Because any deterioration in the child's condition will increase his metabolic needs and could compromise his cerebral perfusion, the nurse or anaesthetist should be able to advise on acceptable ranges for intracranial-pressure and blood pressure measurements; cerebral-perfusion pressure may also need to be monitored during the procedures/interventions. It is sometimes necessary to position the child to control the intracranial pressure – a standard position being 30 degrees head tilted upwards; this will limit both the ability to undertake, and effectiveness of, postural drainage, i.e: positioning the child to drain specific areas of the lung.

Manual hyperventilation using an anaesthetic bagging circuit can be effective in helping to stimulate a cough and expand areas of atelectasis; however, this should be used minimally as it can increase intracranial pressure and alter the systemic blood pressure (Burns and Paratz 1993).

Humidification for non-intubated patients or saline instilled via the endotracheal tube in intubated patients may be required to help loosen thick secretions and nebulized bronchodilating drugs may be needed to relieve bronchospasm.

If the child has long-term ventilatory needs, a tracheostomy may need to be performed rather than continuing ventilatory support through a nasal or oral endotracheal tube, to prevent the development of laryngeal or subglottic stenosis (narrowing of the upper airway).

Orthopaedic complications

Fractures in the patient with a head injury should be managed with a view to early mobilization of joints, and, when appropriate, early weight-bearing to allow appropriate positioning to be commenced.

Stable pelvic fractures are managed with bed rest. The child is usually nursed in supine, rotation is minimized and sitting is gradually introduced. Mobilization is usually attempted early, i.e; two weeks post-fracture. Unstable pelvic fractures are less commonly seen and are usually treated with external fixation or preferably pelvic traction. Sitting and mobilization begin gradually once there is union of the fracture site.

A femoral fracture, depending on stability, may be treated with traction;

however, this may not be tolerated as the child may be confused or agitated (because of the brain injury) and he may then need internal or external fixation. Fixation will also allow for weight bearing at an earlier stage. The method of immobilizing below-knee fractures will depend upon the stability of the fracture site, using either internal or external fixation or plaster of paris casting. External fixation would be the treatment of choice if there is extensive skin damage or if the fracture is compound whereas internal fixation will be used for a closed unstable fracture. For stable fractures the leg may be manipulated under anaesthetic and a plaster of paris cast applied. These children are initially non-weightbearing, progressing to partial weight-bearing when there is sufficient callus formation.

In our experience, upper-limb fractures are not as common, but usually involve the clavicle, scapula, and the neck of humerus. Generally these are stable and do not require surgical intervention. They can be mobilized within the limits of pain. Lower motor neurone damage, for example brachial plexus injury, is relatively uncommon but must be considered during the initial assessment and treated appropriately.

Physical assessment

Whilst ventilated, the child may be paralysed which masks any underlying abnormal postural tone and prevents the assessment of tone. As soon as paralysing agents are reduced and withdrawn, physical assessment of postural tone, the degree of voluntary movement present, and the child's patterns of movement can then be more accurately assessed.

Initially, postural muscle tone is frequently high and usually involves the entire body. There is often a predominance of flexor spasticity in the upper limbs with increased extensor tone in the lower limbs. The presence of extensor thrust may cause the patient to arch his back, extending his head and neck. In supine, this may cause him to become opisthotonic, i.e; arching and lifting his trunk off the bed, and when supported in standing it may cause him to push backwards, his whole body becoming rigid. This severe spasticity does not necessarily persist for longer than the initial few weeks, but needs to be managed appropriately as muscle contractures and subsequent joint deformities can develop rapidly. The joints most likely to be involved are ankles into plantarflexion, and elbows and wrists into flexion. All joints need to be monitored whenever possible by moving the limbs passively through their range of motion. In the presence of very increased muscle tone and abnormal postures, e.g. the child with arms held tightly into his chest, passive movements may not be possible or appropriate. This will be better managed by inhibition of increased tone through careful positioning and inhibitory movements.

Assessment of tone and postural patterns involves evaluating the child in supine, sidelying, prone, and, if possible, sitting and standing. Subsequently, a positioning programme is agreed with the nursing staff and play specialists, using the positions which least encourage spasticity and hopefully allow the child to relax; this can then be continued throughout the day. Tolerance to handling and positioning is variable, and where a child is irritable the programme has to be tailored to his level of tolerance. As with all management, reassessment should occur at each session and is particularly important at this time as change in physical status can occur rapidly.

Splintage

Plastazote resting splints are the most commonly used type to maintain the length of the achilles tendons and elbow flexors; in the presence of very high tone, serial splinting may be required. The splints should be worn intermittently throughout the day, increasing the length of time within the child's tolerance, and also at night if possible. Close attention should be made to the skin as pressure marks can quickly appear, particularly if the child has altered consciousness or a sensory deficit.

Plastering (often serially) of the ankles and elbows is an alternative to splinting; one obvious disadvantage to plastering is the inability to have hydrotherapy if this facility is available.

Role of occupational therapy

The early treatment phase allows the therapist to sit and talk to parents/ carers and to learn as much as possible about the child's lifestyle, interests/ likes and dislikes/friends/ brothers and sisters etc. In order to engage the child's co-operation and motivation, these ideas will form the media through which the occupational therapist will later work.

The occupational therapist will work with the family, set realistic aims and objectives for treatment, in ways which are meaningful to the child's needs and desires. From this point it is essential to liaise and also work closely with the physiotherapist and speech therapist in order to combine facilitation of good quality of movement or language production through valued activities.

In the early stages, part of the overall rehabilitation objective is to increase the child's level of sensory awareness which will clearly contribute to his physical recovery. A multisensory approach is desirable with a combination of olfactory, tactile, auditory, and visual stimulation. The child's reactions are carefully monitored and the degree and depth of awareness are noted. Olfactory recognition is important in its own right and also in its relation to taste. One or two strong smells are introduced in addition to explanation and timing of response. These should be items familiar to the child, e.g. chocolate, peppermint, orange or coffee.

Tactile stimulation is assessed to identify whether the child has reduced sensation or hypersensitivity to touch by providing graded stimuli, from heavy to light pressure, combinations of hot and cold etc. The occupational therapist must be aware of the possible effect of tactile stimulation on the overall postural tone ie, stimulation may increase already high muscle tone, and also of tactile defensiveness ie, an 'over reaction' of the child's sensory receptors to stimulation.

When assessing auditory awareness it is necessary to focus the child's attention on single sounds in a quiet background. Although there are commercially available tapes of everyday home and school sounds, tapes of friends, family and familiar music are encouraged. Parents are encouraged to talk to the child as they previously did (even though initially they may not get much response) giving news of home, family, and daily events.

If the child appears to have visual difficulties it is clearly important to formally assess and regularly monitor visual responses. If still in bed, position the child's head supported on a wedge cushion. Initially establish the child's ability to visually fixate upon, for example, a single bright object. Monitor their eye movements in all visual planes in response to this stimulus. Ask parents how much they feel that their child is seeing, for both near and far distance. At this stage advise the parents regarding positioning of toys at approximately shoulder level, using natural light from behind the child (or supplementary artificial light), or identify any particular colours to which the child responds. This approach should be used as a starting point in gaining their visual attention.

In the early stage of rehabilitiation these sessions should remain brief, as the child may only have short periods of full consciousness; in addition, even when awake, his concentration or attention span may also be very limited.

INTERMEDIATE REHABILITATION

Physical presentation

Physical presentation is obviously variable, depending upon the site and extent of brain damage. From our experience, the most common outcome is hemiplegia, but quadriplegia, ataxia, and dyskinesias are also common. Not uncommonly, there may be a combination of these deficits (Scott-Jupp *et al* 1992). The combination of hemiplegia and ataxia usually presents with ataxia on the opposite side to the hemiplegia. This is because the corticospinal tracts cross in the brainstem, causing spasticity on the opposite side to the lesion, whereas cerebellar damage causes ataxia on the same side as the lesion. When postural tone is initially very high, ataxia may not be obvious until the tone has decreased and active movement then becomes possible; as the child's ability to move improves and range of movement increases, it may even appear as though the ataxia is increasing.

An uncommon presentation is athetoid hemiplegia, which is manifest by the development of fluctuating tone and frequent, involuntary (uncontrolled) writhing movements; these movements may interfere significantly with functional activities (e.g. dressing, eating, and writing), often persist and are usually poorly controlled with drugs.

Muscle tone

Assessment of postural tone involves consideration of factors such as irritability, level of consciousness, sensory problems, as well as the level of understanding which will alter basic tone. Spasticity may be increased (often markedly so) if the child is still irritable or fearful, or if he is in pain, although this can be difficult to appreciate if communication is limited. As the child starts to become more aware, frustration can also increase his tone.

With acquired brain injury, spasticity does not always occur in similar patterns that are seen with children with cerebral palsy. It is possible to see isolated increased tone, e.g. spasticity in the shoulder girdle with increased flexor tone in the elbow, but little or no increase in flexor tone in the hand.

Muscle tone may be assessed using passive movements and by observing how the child moves from one position to another. If resistance to certain movements is felt or observed, the cause for this can then be identified. When the child starts to move, associated reactions may be seen, i.e. any voluntary movement performed with effort may cause an increase in spasticity in another part. These associated movements must be closely monitored as they can contribute to the development of contractures and deformities by accentuating the patterns of spasticity (Bobath and Bobath 1984). If the child uses abnormal patterns to move, it will further increase any abnormal muscle tone. Involuntary (ataxic or athetoid) movements can also become more marked as the activity of the child increases.

Muscle relaxants, including baclofen, dantrolene, L-DOPA, and diazepam are often required in the early stages to reduce severe levels of spasticity to a more 'manageable' level. Close discussion is necessary with the medical staff to decide on the optimum doses. It is clearly important to review the need for these drugs regularly as the child's muscle tone and any associated involuntary movements resolve – or plateau. In the case of severe degrees of focal (localized) spasticity (e.g. affecting the elbow and forearm flexors), intramuscular injections of botulinum toxin may be used; in our experience, this has produced encouraging results although occasionally repeated injections have been required to maintain the initial benefit. Botulinum toxin provides a temporary reduction in tone to the individual muscle or muscle group injected, which should be reinforced with regular physiotherapy post-injection.

Assessment of sensation

In the early stages it is usually possible, during handling and treatment sessions, to gain an overall impression of obvious sensory loss and/or neglect as well as hypersensitivity to touch or to textures. However, formal testing of sensation in the brain injured child can be difficult. Guidance from the speech therapist will be required regarding the child's level of understanding of language; for example, will he be able to understand 'hot' and 'cold' (He also needs to have sufficient expressive language or some means of communicating a response by a symbol or sign, for example, to respond if he can feel that he is being touched). If the child has expressive problems if may not be possible to ask him to name an object in a test of stereognosis and it may have to be structured, eg by asking 'is this a brush or a pen'.

Aims of treatment

The overall aim is to assist and, hopefully, enable the child to achieve and regain maximum independence following the brain injury.

Broadly, the conjoint aims of physiotherapy and occupational therapy are to:

- position to restore and maintain alignment
- prevent contractures and deformities
- normalize postural tone and facilitate normal movement
- increase sensory awareness
- increase balance reactions and restore alignment
- facilitate self-help skills and establish broad perceptual abilities.

Although a number of these objectives will fall within the principal responsibility of either the physiotherapist or the occupational therapist, it is obvious that there will be common areas and objectives, again stressing the need for a multidisciplinary liaison and treatment plan, and joint-therapy sessions. It is also clear that as the child progresses through the rehabilitation programme and demonstrates increasing recovery, the objectives – and therefore the therapists' input – will change, focusing more on the child's functional and educational abilities.

Principles of treatment

Our approach is based on the principles of neurodevelopmental treatment. The prior-learned normal movement can accelerate the rehabilitation process. This is unlike cerebral palsy where even an *in utero* experience is likely to be already impaired (Bryce 1976).

In the brain injured child, spasticity usually occurs due to damage to the cerebral cortex, and produces a lack of inhibition from the higher centres.

Inhibition of abnormal postural tone through handling counteracts abnormal tone and patterns of posture and movement. Normal patterns of movement are dependent on normal postural tone. It is impossible to superimpose normal movement onto a background of abnormal postural tone. Physiotherapy should aim to give the child (who has the potential to move) more normal patterns of movement; facilitation of such movement makes active motor responses possible (Bryce 1972)

The key to successful treatment is through careful handling. In treatment sessions, the child should not be allowed to perform movements and activities in abnormal ways using abnormal postural tone. Through controlled activity the child experiences the sensation of more normal movement and there should therefore be constant feedback between the child and the therapist. Use of repetition of movement will help the child to relearn movements. It is important to handle the child minimally and hand over control of the movement to the child.

It has been shown that the injured developing brain has an amazing capacity to reorganize its growth connections whilst they are still being formed. The concept of rehabilitation based on neurodevelopmental treatment (i.e. relearning normal movement by inhibiting abnormal tone and movement and facilitating normal activity) is reinforced physiologically with these ideas of neuromuscular plasticity. These ideas rely on the fact that the nervous system is able to adapt to changes forced upon it during development and during recovery from disease and injury. Physiologically, it has been shown that in order for a child with an acquired brain injury to be rehabilitated to his full potential, plastic changes within the brain which enhance normal movement must be encouraged. If abnormal movement is allowed it will become reinforced and the central nervous system will adapt to these abnormal movements, allowing them to become established; this will, in turn, decrease function. According to the theories of neuroplasticity the physiological aims of therapy are therefore:

- strengthening normal synaptic chains and neuronal sets
- guiding axonal sprouting
- facilitating unmasking of alternative or previously unused pathways in the central nervous system
- maintaining normal function through alternate routes.

The facilitation of normal movement should strengthen and maintain muscles for functional tasks. It should also reduce the spasticity through the opening of pathways for normal movement (Kidd *et al.* 1992).

These ideas support theoretically what physiotherapy has been claiming to achieve practically for many years. Occasionally, misconnections due to spurious synapses can transmit disruptive information and unbalance normal information (Kidd *et al.* 1992), and in these situations, plasticity of the central nervous system is therefore not always desirable!

Depending on the child's physical problems, treatment is aimed at improving head and trunk control which enables sitting balance to be achieved. Firstly, the child should be able to hold his head statically in alignment, then move his head in isolation from his body by moving out of alignment and correcting back into alignment, i.e. head and trunk-righting reactions. The child needs head control for eating, communication, orientation in space, and paying attention to what is happening around him. Balance will improve as postural tone is normalized and as the child begins to move using more normal patterns of movement; initially, this will focus on sitting balance, but subsequently on standing and, hopefully, walking.

Children with ataxia will have problems with coordination. This is due to poor proximal stability, which if improved with treatment, can help to reduce the influence of the ataxia.

A child who is disorientated may have problems with motor planning, which impedes his ability to sequence movements. Such sequences may have to be retaught using repetition, initially breaking down the movements into smaller sequences which he will remember with practice, e.g. when moving from lying to sitting, the child may need to practise rolling from supine into sidelying, and moving from sidelying into sitting over the side of the bed by pushing through his arms. The child may be slow at understanding and processing this information and it is therefore important to give him plenty of time to respond to instructions.

If the child has spent a considerable length of time on the ICU there may be true muscle weakness. However, when abnormal tone is present, muscle weakness should be regarded as a secondary problem. The function of some muscles will be affected by abnormal co-contraction, e.g. lack of ability to extend the elbow due to flexor spasticity in elbow flexors. Once the high postural tone has been reduced generally and functional activity returned, this weakness may no longer be a problem. If true weakness still exists then this can be addressed using stimulatory techniques such as tapping and sweeping, although these techniques should be used with caution if increased tone persists.

General issues

The overall aim is to try and achieve the maximum potential of the child's ability – physically, cognitively, and emotionally. To be effective, the physiotherapist and occupational therapist must work closely with the play specialist, speech and language therapist, and the child's family, setting joint aims of treatment. Joint therapy sessions are useful to incorporate appropriate positioning with functional activity. It is important to understand that as the child's rehabilitation proceeds there will be an increasing number of different therapy sessions that the child must attend; this may initially confuse the child, which may be avoided or at least reduced by holding joint sessions. Additionally, extreme fatigue will impinge upon the child's performance, and so he will achieve most if therapy time can be provided in concise sessions. Speech therapy advice regarding the child's level of understanding is essential to enable the therapists and ward staff to use instructions appropriately (Hall et al. 1990). Ensuring that all involved with the child's care and rehabilitation programme have the same understanding and objectives will maximise the child's potential for recovery.

As soon as the child's individual rehabilitiation programme has been established, a weekly timetable is agreed to co-ordinate daily therapies. Rest periods should be included for the child who fatigues and tires very easily. Posture and control of movement deteriorates with fatigue, which is a particular problem in a child with ataxia.

The number of physiotherapy and occupational sessions will obviously vary depending upon the severity of the child's brain injury, 'needs', and the stage of his rehabilitation programme. It is essential for the success of any treatment plan and regime to be communicated to, and undertaken in conjunction with, the ward staff and parents, for example correct positioning for lying in bed, sitting with appropriate support, or periods of standing in a standing frame. This will facilitate regular positional changes which, by bringing the child up against gravity, may help to raise the child's level of consciousness and overall orientation. Carers should also be aware of the length of time that the child should remain in each position, as a child who has little or no active movement will soon become stiff and uncomfortable which may further increase abnormal postural tone as well as increasing their fatigue. Such children will also be a greater risk of contractures and deformities developing if they are left in a position for too long. Advice will also be required on how to handle the child when changing their position, e.g. transferring from chair to bed, etc.

A limiting factor, particularly in the early stages of treatment, may be aggression, irritability, drowsiness, or fatigue. The child may be very fearful of being handled, particularly if they have visual problems, a hearing deficit or other sensory problems. It is therefore crucial to handle the child slowly and with care, introducing position changes gradually. A simple and often repeated explanation of what you plan to do may help to calm the child, and is good practice, even when the child is unconscious or is thought to have impaired vision or hearing. If a child does not appear to tolerate a position even for a short period of time, it may be that it is too soon to introduce that position, or it may require modification; e.g. if sitting upright is not tolerated, the child may need to adjust to reclined sitting first. If the child does become aggressive or his behaviour is inappropriate when being handled, then this should be discouraged whilst good behaviour should be praised. Behaviour modification techniques are frequently required and advice on when and how these techniques are implemented is provided by the clinical psychologist member of the team.

Initially, the child may cry for prolonged periods, particularly when being handled in therapy sessions. Parents who are obviously very upset by the devastating and sudden change which has occurred to their child may find this hard to cope with and question the therapist about the necessity of the specific therapy or, rarely, ask to terminate the therapy session. Reassurance is often required that their child is not in pain when being handled and that the crying will eventually settle. Initially some parents may find attending therapy sessions too difficult as it highlights the physical difficulties the child now has, and this should be respected; in this situation, parents should be gradually introduced to the ideas behind, and reasons for doing, the therapy. Other parents may try to cope by constantly working with the child on the ideas given by the therapists, and these parents need to be reminded that the child needs to have planned and regular periods of rest throughout the day.

Positioning and ideas for treatment

Once medically stable and breathing spontaneously, the child may be able to start sitting with support, although this may initially be for very short periods. At this point, supported standing can also be commenced. If the child has a significant degree of distal extensor spasticity, it is important to introduce standing as soon as possible as an inhibitory position or 'technique' to prevent the development of contractures of the achilles tendons.

It is important to assess the child in each position, looking at his postural tone (at rest and under stimulation), the symmetry of the child's position, and the ability of the child to adapt and accept the position, in order to advise carers on a positioning programme which can be followed on the ward.

Lying Lying is a very supportive position and, as the base of support is large, no balance is required to maintain this position.

1. *Supine* (i.e. lying face upwards) is recognized to be a position which increases extensor tone, if extensor spasticity is present. Initially, the child may present with a predominant pattern of extensor spasticity with flexor spasticity in upper limbs, i.e. arching backwards of head with extension of the neck, retraction of scapulae (usually accompanied by protraction and adduction of the shoulders and flexor pattern in the arms), extension and adduction in the legs with plantarflexion in the feet. It is important to check whether the child is pushing into the surface with the back of his head or his elbows or heels as this extensor spasticity may increase when the child is positioned in the supine position. If so, this position should be avoided or modified, e.g. the use of a neck cushion or wedge to elongate the neck and to introduce flexion into the hips with use of a pillow under the knees to introduce a small amount of flexion into the legs.

Ideas for treatment. Supine is a good position to work on leg control initially, as the patient is fully supported. If spasticity is present in either or both legs, control of leg movements into extension and flexion can be developed without spasticity taking over the movement. The foot should be held in dorsiflexion, and the leg assisted to move from flexion to extension without the foot pushing down or rotation occurring in the hips. The patient can gradually take the weight of his limb, working into a greater range of flexion and extension as his control improves (Figs 5.1 and 5.2).

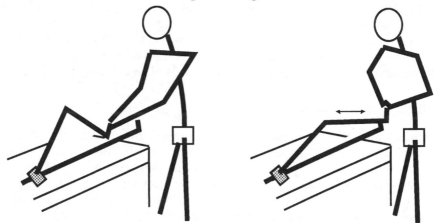

Figs. 5.1 and 5.2   Assisting control of leg movements into flexion and extension

A variation of supine is crook-lying, when the knees are flexed and the feet placed flat on the bed. In this position, isolated pelvic control can be gained, particularly lifting the pelvis into extension which is good preparation for antigravity control when standing. In a child with hemiplegia, weight-bearing can be encouraged over the affected side by lifting the sound foot off the bed whilst maintaining the position of the pelvis and affected leg (Figs 5.3 and 5.4).

2. *Prone* (i.e. lying face downwards) is recognized to be a position which increases flexor tone. It is therefore a useful position to use with children with a predominance of extensor tone who need to avoid lying supine. It appears to be a successful position for settling children who are still quite agitated and do not settle easily in bed.

Ideas for treatment. Some children, particularly those with visual problems, may need to be prepared prior to positioning in prone, i.e. work on rolling, gradually taking the child into the prone position. It may need to be modified slightly to increase his comfort, i.e. as he is positioned over a wedge, the legs may relax into flexion at the knee with support to the lower leg, which will help to break up the extensor pattern in the legs. The head can be left unsupported which allows for neck elongation, or rotated and rested on a pillow, although care needs to be taken in preventing asymmetry developing throughout the trunk. A preference for turning the head to one side may indicate that asymmetry is already present, in terms of increased postural tone in one side of the body. The arms should be placed in an elevated position over the wedge, if possible, to maintain the joint range in the shoulders and allow scapular movement. This may require preparation, e.g. firstly work in prone over a gym ball, and careful handling if the child has been or is very stiff (Fig 5.5).

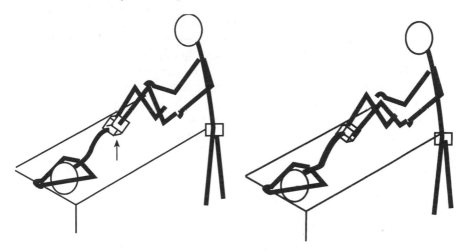

Figs. 5.3 and 5.4 Crook-lying for pelvic control

Smaller children can be positioned over a parent's, nurse's, or another therapist's lap; this allows movement to be introduced by gently rocking the person's legs. Pelvic rotation can also be introduced to inhibit increased tone.

Prone can be used when treatment is progressing as it encourages extensor activity in the head and upper trunk. This can be performed on a wedge or, if movement is required, on a roll or therapy ball. Prone is also a good position to develop weight transference in the arms, freeing one arm whilst weightbearing on the other. This can usually be incorporated into well disguised "play" sessions, by engaging the child in games which encourage head lifting and/ or one handed use, thus promoting practice of good positioning through a medium of meaningful and 'interesting' activities.

3. *Sidelying* is a useful position as it is a midposition between supine and prone, with predominance of extension of the weight-bearing side and flexion of the non-weight-bearing side; however, a child with strong extensor thrust

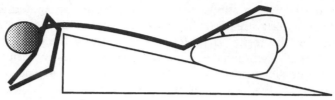

Fig. 5.5   Lying prone on a wedge.

initiated from their head may predominantly extend in this position. Advantages of using sidelying are to elongate the weight-bearing side, improve alignment of the head on the body (which will help with midline orientation), and enabling the hands to come together and also to the face and mouth to increase body awareness. The disadvantage of sidelying is that the base of support is less than in supine or prone; the child may feel less safe and therefore distressed in this position, which may cause an increase in their postural tone. A child with hemiplegia who has poor proprioception and decreased cutaneous sensation on their affected side may become particularly unsettled when placed on this side.

Ideas for treatment. Sidelying is a good position to use in joint-therapy sessions when starting to re-develop mid-line orientation, visual regard of both hands and early hand eye co-ordination. Activities should be age appropriate for the child and should be graded to enable him to succeed.

Movement in and out of sidelying requires the ability to combine flexion and extension through rotation. As treatment progresses, sidelying can be used to combine activity of flexion and extension, working towards dissociation of movement of trunk and limbs. Sidelying is an important position when the child starts to move, particularly when changing position from lying to sitting.

Rolling   When learning to roll between supine and prone, the child has to move through sidelying. Facilitation of rolling in and out of sidelying, using rotation between the shoulder girdle and pelvis, may be effective in inhibiting increased tone. In a child with hemiplegia, rolling towards the affected side will also increase awareness of this side. When learning to roll towards his unaffected side the child should be encouraged to clasp both hands together, reach the arms into extension, and rotate from the upper trunk, moving both arms together towards the sound side, the legs following, with assistance if necessary.

Sitting   Sitting requires, and uses, a combination of patterns of flexion (hips and knees) and extension (trunk and head). The base of support is less than in lying, requiring some ability to balance against gravity. This requires good interplay of the muscles within the trunk. Sitting unsupported independently also requires a degree of alertness; therefore a child with even a mild head injury may initially require support to maintain a sitting position if he is drowsy and disorientated.

Ideas for treatment. Sitting balance may need to be developed initially with support by weight-bearing through extended arms. It is desirable in a child with a hemiplegia to facilitate weight-bearing over the affected side by sitting on his affected side, placing the hand onto the bed and supporting the shoulder under the axilla (armpit), whilst slowly assisting the child to weight-shift over his affected side and elongating the trunk at the same time (Fig 5.6).

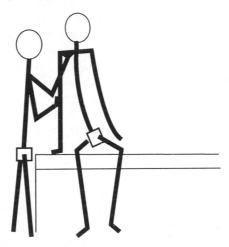

Fig. 5.6 Weight bearing over the affected side with trunk elongation.

Children with a predominance of extensor spasticity are difficult to position in sitting and may not tolerate the position for long due to the flexion introduced to their hips and knees. In a child with extensor thrust initiated from the head, it may be necessary to elongate the neck to inhibit this, and the hips will need to be maintained in at least 90 degrees of flexion, sometimes more, to inhibit the extensor tone in the legs. It is possible to achieve this position in younger children whilst supported on a therapist's or carer's knee, but older children may need two people or a supportive chair to achieve and maintain a sitting position. If the feet are in contact with a surface they should be placed in neutral and may need to be held in this position to inhibit pushing into plantarflexion due to extensor tone. Sometimes the plinth or footplate may need to be raised to prevent the child pushing into extension.

If the child has a predominance of increased flexor tone in his upper trunk causing a pull into flexion, this should be inhibited using trunk rotation, then active extension of the lumbar spine facilitated. In some cases it may be necessary to prepare the child for sitting, e.g. first working in standing with appropriate support, which will encourage extensor activity, and then progressing to develop a good sitting posture. An ataxic or low-toned child may need to develop increased proximal stability to maintain his balance, using techniques such as compression through the trunk or tapping. The child will gain trunk control gradually, therefore support can be gradually lowered down to their pelvis as control is gained proximally.

As the child starts to develop static and dynamic sitting balance, he is in one of the optimum positions in which to make meaningful sense of the visual, auditory, tactile and olfactory information in the environment. The child's ability to translate this into an internal schema (or perceptual ability) can be assessed skilfully through the media of games and activities. For example, by observing the child's responses during a card game of 'pairs' the occupational therapist can start to evaluate the child's thought processing skills, visual discriminatory skills, ability to remember and follow directions, length of concentration span, short-term visual memory and ability to attend to material presented. If the task presented is matched to the interests of the child or provides him with a novel approach (which is both inviting and fun), any activity can be carefully used as a treatment media. Assessment takes the form of observation, the most important point to note is *how* a child approaches and executes a task. To the skilled therapist this will provide a clue to the child's underlying abilities and disabilities.

Once the child starts to achieve dynamic sitting balance, practice of previously learned functional skills can resume. Advantage can be taken of this position, to promote active participation in activities of daily living, such as dressing, washing, eating, drinking etc. According to the child's physical abilities and inabilities, therapists can discuss the child's readiness for participation in such activities and can teach parents/carers ways in which to carry out the activities which will maximise and promote good quality of the necessary physical movements, whilst at the same time providing realistic and meaningful goals for the child, through media which are familiar and realistic. For example, for the child with asymmetry who is to learn to dress his top half, the activity can be modified therapeutically. If the child exhibits visual neglect in one half of his field of vision, he must always be encouraged to dress with a table in front of him. This is for three reasons: i) it enables a garment to be laid out correctly, thus limiting confusion caused by poor spatial judgement or poor recognition of concepts such as front/back/inside out etc., ii) it provides an opportunity for the child to visually regard the whole garment and to look over to a neglected side of his body and iii) it provides a stable surface from which the child can work.

The child is taught to position his less functional arm in extension across the table so that he has every opportunity to remember that it exists. He is then taught to always dress this arm first, using his functional arm to ease on clothes and adjust them accordingly. If possible, the child can be encouraged to link his hands together to assist with easing tops over his head. Finally he is taught to check with his functional hand that clothing on both sides of his body is adjusted evenly.

The child will initially achieve static balance, followed by movement in sitting which can be encouraged by weight transference, introducing trunk rotation, and reaching outside the base of support, all of which require reliable equilibrium reactions. When trying to develop sitting balance, one technique, using reciprocal activity of all the trunk muscles, would be to place the child on a mobile surface such as a roll or ball. The child needs to respond quickly with graded movements using equilibrium reactions and trunk-righting reactions to maintain midline orientation. This is particularly useful in children with proximal instability. Slow rhythmical movements can be effective at inhibiting increased flexor tone, particularly in children with hemiplegia who use the spasticity to fixate and balance. Introducing rotation in sitting will also help to inhibit flexor spasticity, but active extension also needs to be established.

The child with any degree of asymmetry should be taught how to move in sitting through the transference of weight to the unaffected side, moving the affected side with assistance if necessary, firstly forwards and backwards and later side to side. This encompasses trunk rotation and weight transference.

A child who has moderate/marked increased muscle tone in his legs commonly finds long periods of sitting an uncomfortable position to maintain, due to tightness in the hamstrings particularly if there is limited pelvic mobility. This can be a good position to develop increasing hamstring length through a prolonged stretch. Adverse neural tension techniques may also be required if the sciatic nerve is involved.

Seating Assessment of the child's seating needs can be difficult. It is impossible to have available every type of seat that may be required, and as the child may change rapidly in his physical presentation (sometimes only requiring specialized seating initially), it is impracticable to order personalized seating until the child's long-term needs can be assessed. Chairs may therefore have to be adapted to suit the child's needs, and obviously these should be reassessed as the child improves. Ideally the child needs both a static chair (for use on the ward, at home, and eventually, if necessary, in school) and wheelchair or buggy.

When considering positioning in sitting it is important to consider the position of the pelvis, as this will influence head and trunk alignment and may alter postural tone distally. The patient should not be allowed to weight-bear through the ischium or 'sacrally sit' as this will affect their sitting balance and overall function. It is important to try and achieve 90 degrees at the hips, knees, and ankles. If distal extensor tone is very high it may be necessary to hold the feet in neutral by using straps at 45 degrees to the ankles, or the sandals provided in some supportive seating, to encourage weight-bearing through the heels. This needs to be carefully monitored to ensure that the child does not push through his feet, further increasing his tone. In such cases, foot support may not be possible until the tone has settled, although the child can wear his plastazote splints to maintain a neutral foot position.

The child may initially require a chair with an extended back or headrest, possibly with side supports, to give sufficient support to the head and neck if he has poor head control. If possible this tilt should not take place at the hips because the hip to trunk angle should be maintained at 90 degrees to limit extensor spasticity. The seat depth should also allow 90 degrees of hip and knee flexion. Ramped cushions can sometimes be useful to increase or decrease the hip to trunk angle if there is a high degree of extensor or flexor spasticity in the hips. Lumbar, waist, and chest supports may also be necessary to maintain correct body alignment. A pommel may be required to maintain hip abduction.

A child with low postural tone will sit with legs falling out into abduction, external rotation at the hip, and supination of the feet. This can be corrected by placing padding between the sides of the chair and the legs to bring the legs together. Some chairs provide sandals on the foot rest which are useful for strapping the feet in a good position. If his trunk is not well supported, he may fall into flexion and side flexion due to poor extensor activity; waistcoats which attach to the chair may be very effective at correcting this.

The wheelchair should have removable foot plates to allow for standing transfers. A wheelchair or buggy will not only provide the child with a means of transport to get to therapy sessions, it will also allow the family a chance to take him out, which may help to calm him if he is agitated or frustrated.

In summary, it is important that the child is seated in a functional position, in a chair in which his trunk is well-supported, his pelvis symmetrical, his feet well-positioned on a footrest, and with head support if necessary.

Standing   Standing is a more total pattern of extension, with extension in hips and knees, but dorsiflexion in ankles. It is therefore frequently the preferred position to try and develop head control than sitting, where there is more influence of flexion.

Methods of standing. Initially, a tilt table or supine standing frame is usually required to provide sufficient support, particularly for those with little or no head control. A prone stander is suitable for children with some head control and an upright stander is suitable for those with good head and some trunk control. Children with less severe head injuries and smaller children can be stood with therapist support. Ensuring alignment is very important when standing these children as they may not yet have sufficient righting reactions to be able to readjust their positioning. In a child with poor trunk control, a standing frame with side trunk support is more suitable than the tilt table in preventing pulling or falling into side flexion if asymmetry is present. If the child has a significant degree of distal extensor spasticity, his feet may remain in plantarflexion when stood, causing him to stand on his toes. This may be gradually inhibited through weight-bearing, allowing the heel to drop into a neutral ankle position. If this does not happen, it may be necessary for the child to wear plastazote splints whilst standing, as shoes may be too difficult to wear. If plantarflexion can be inhibited, but the feet become inverted, wearing aircast splints will help to control this in the short term. When the postural tone is very high, extensor spasticity may also cause the knees to hyperextend in standing. In the tilt table or supine stander this should be controlled by placing a small roll behind the knees. A roll may also be required between the legs to maintain some abduction. If the frame has a tray this will allow for weight-bearing through the forearms. This is also a good position for the play specialists to work with the child, which has the added advantage of distracting the child if he is not happy in the frame.

Some centres prefer not to use tilt tables as the child remains extended when being moved from lying to standing, which is not a normal movement sequence. An additional disadvantage of using a tilt table or standing frame is that the child may be more passive than when being stood between two therapists. However, the tilt table does allow the child to learn to adjust to a standing position and stand in a corrected position for longer periods, thereby enabling inhibitory weight-bearing as well as a prolonged stretch to the achilles tendons. Providing that standing balance and control of sitting to standing is commenced at the appropriate time, it is our experience that no long term problems are caused by inclined standing on a supine stander or tilt table.

An alternative method to standing the child with support may be to use a therapy ball, on which the child can be placed in prone lying and gradually brought upright into a standing position. This can be a useful method for an agitated child who cannot tolerate any one position for very long, as his position can be quickly readjusted from prone lying to standing within his level of tolerance.

Ideas for treatment. Initially, standing balance may be achieved using support to arms and upper body, possibly resting at 90 degrees onto a plinth; this will then allow the physiotherapist to facilitate weight transference between the right and left leg. When attempting to progress to sequencing from sitting to standing it is important to ensure the feet are parallel and the child weight-bears through both feet equally. A child with sensory problems may benefit if pressure is applied through the knee on the affected side to reinforce symmetry and the sensation of weight bearing. The child needs to be guided to lean forwards with his upper body in alignment, particularly if extensor tone still predominates (and vice versa for standing to sitting). This sequence can be broken down to small ranges when trying to develop proximal stability in the pelvis, which is useful when poor coactivation is a problem, e.g. children with ataxia.

If supported standing is too difficult for the child to achieve, prone standing will provide more support to the upper body, i.e. resting head and trunk onto a plinth with hips at 90 degrees whilst weight-bearing through legs.

Ladderback chairs can be useful for support with smaller children – particularly those with poor proximal stability, including ataxia – who can hold onto a bar for assistance but need to work hard in their trunk and pelvis to maintain balance in standing. Compression and tapping can be used proximally to increase this activity.

Gradually, as standing balance improves, support should be reduced until the child can stand unsupported. Sometimes, as support is being reduced to allow the child to take control, a tall stick for one or both hands can be used which will assist with balance without allowing the child to lean. If distal extensor tone remains difficult to inhibit, the child may benefit from ankle foot orthoses (known as AFOs), depending upon the distribution of tone.

Once symmetry in standing with equal weight-bearing has been achieved, the patient should work on weight transference, which is a prerequisite for stepping. A progression of standing is step-standing where one foot is forwards from the other. This will reduce the base of support and is a harder position to maintain balance. Again, weight transfer should be established in preparation for walking. In a child with hemiplegia, placing the affected leg behind will require the ability to dorsiflex beyond 90 degrees at the ankle as the weight is transferred onto the front leg; this sequence is obviously required to achieve gait and ambulation. When the affected leg is forwards the ankle will be in slight plantarflexion which would require the patient to overcome any distal extensor tone. Working from standing to step-standing via stepping requires reliable balance reactions of the supporting leg, which necessitates some hip and knee control and the ability to place the moving leg. If hip or knee control remains poor the therapist can support the area or the patient can use the plinth closely behind him, gradually reducing the support as control improves (Fig 5.7).

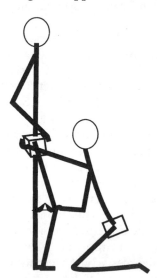

Fig. 5.7 Working for hip and knee control in standing.

A wobble-board can be useful to refine balance for a child who has reasonable standing balance. The child is required to respond by counter-balancing to changes in external forces as the wobble-board moves. This requires reliable, graded balance reactions and constant feedback through proprioception to maintain alignment. Care should be taken if the child still has some spasticity as postural tone may increase if the speed or range of movement of the board is too great for the child to balance. A progression, once balance has been achieved, is to teach the child to throw and catch a ball whilst maintaining their balance on the board (Fig 5.8).

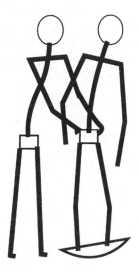

Fig. 5.8 Working to improve balance on a 'wobble board'.

One-legged standing is a position requiring a great deal of balance; however, it may be important to develop one-legged balance if the child is returning to mainstream school and to full participation in sporting activities. It can be developed initially by placing one foot on a ball, therefore shifting the weight onto the other leg. This can also be a good position for developing knee control into extension of the predominantly weight-bearing leg. A child with balance problems can also be taught strategies such as visually fixing on a static object at eye level.

Standing provides an excellent position for the occupational therapist and physiotherapist to work together to optimise good functional positioning. The child is well placed to develop and use his skills of perception, sensory awareness, proprioception and kinaesthetic awareness. Through the use of games, quizzes etc. the child's cognitive abilities in terms of short and long term memory, recall of previously learned skills, thought processing and problem solving strategies for new skills, can begin to be ascertained. By using this approach, the child will probably only be aware of the 'fun' element of participating and will generally co-operate well in response. An example of this may be the use of a popular 'Four in a Row' game, which the child may well be familiar with.

Walking   An obvious and often crucial goal for the child and his family is walking. However, it is important that the child should be ready for this, which sometimes requires a great deal of patience from the child and family – and from the medical and nursing staff! If standing balance is poor, with reduced equilibrium reactions, it is not beneficial to practise walking with the assistance of a therapist or nursing staff before the child is ready, as it is likely to frighten the patient, decreasing his confidence and probably exacerbating any pre-existing spasticity. As a learning experience, early walking without control of the movement does not contribute any kind of useful information to the child's brain (Lynch and Grisogono 1991).

Ideas for treatment. Walking can be facilitated if the child has sufficient standing balance as well as the ability to transfer weight. It begins by stepping sideways against a high plinth, with support through the arms.

When supporting a child with a hemiplegia as he is walking, the therapist or nurse should be on his affected side to assist with balance and movement of the hemiplegic leg and controlling the knee to prevent hyperextension if necessary. Initially, the child should not be given a tripod, quadrapod, or stick as this will increase any asymmetry. A high stick or sticks may be useful later for balance only, and not to weight-bear.

A child with poor proximal stability may benefit initially from intermittent compression down through the pelvis throughout the gait cycle (Fig 5.9). As the child progresses, gait should be facilitated from the upper limbs to ensure activity of the pelvis.

The feet are the main area of movement for balance during the gait cycle, i.e. forwards (plantarflexor activity), backwards (dorsiflexor activity), and sideways (invertor/evertor activity).

If the child has a significant degree of distal extensor tone, dorsiflexor and evertor activity may be impaired which will make balance difficult; in such cases, specific work on these muscle groups may be required to redress the muscle balance. The child should continue to wear the plastazote splints at night, and possibly an AFO for part of, or throughout, the day to maintain the ankle in a neutral position, thus inhibiting extensor tone. With long-term problems, trophic stimulation may be effective, if used appropriately, in increasing activity in these muscles.

Even if a child is beginning to achieve walking in physiotherapy sessions, but is still unsteady, it should be made clear to the child and all who care for him that he is not yet ready to walk around the ward; an effective way of communicating this is to leave clear instructions regarding the child's mobility above his bed!

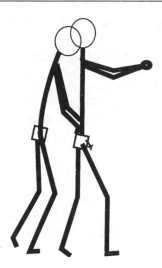

Fig. 5.9   Facilitation of walking from the pelvis.

A tricycle is a useful alternative method of mobility in smaller children which allows a degree of independence; it also encourages bilateral arm support, which is beneficial for children with hemiplegia and also those who have dissociation of lower limbs. A child with ataxia who is unsteady may benefit by using a Kaye-walker for support; push along trucks can be used for smaller children.

Hydrotherapy

Hydrotherapy may be valuable, particularly in the early period of rehabilitation when it may be difficult to inhibit tone and settle the child effectively.

The warmth of the water (approximately 36°C) combined with the use of inhibitory techniques will help to relieve increased muscle tone. Total immersion for a period of 15–20 minutes has been shown to relieve spasticity (Martin 1983). This is extremely useful in allowing increased joint range when tone is too high to permit passive movements.

Inhibitory techniques such as 'snaking' can be used i.e. using the drag of the water to facilitate elongation of the side flexors of the trunk, and introducing rotation as necessary to inhibit spasticity proximally and therefore achieve relaxation distally. This can be an extremely effective way to relax and calm the child. As postural tone is often closely related to the child's emotional status, reduction of tone may be achieved more successfully in water. In our experience this is particularly true when the child was a keen swimmer prior to sustaining the brain injury.

The hydrotherapy pool is a good place to introduce the feeling of normal movement in a child who has restricted movements, and can be used for preparation for movement on dry land, e.g. facilitating horizontal rotation in water to encourage rolling on land.

The treatment plan for hydrotherapy is planned in liaison with the 'land' therapist and would be similar to the child's 'land' treatment. The hydrotherapist may find that balance in sitting and standing is more easily achieved because of the buoyancy and support of the water. Sequences of movement, such as sitting to standing and walking, may also be greatly assisted and facilitated by buoyancy.

A child with a severe brain injury who will never achieve walking may find that he is able to move with more freedom in water. With such children, hydrotherapy can be very rewarding and enjoyable. They can be taught to swim which will allow them a degree of freedom that they no longer have on land. However, this movement may be at the expense of quality, and they should therefore be carefully assessed and monitored to ensure that any active movement they have on land does not deteriorate.

STANDARDIZED ASSESSMENT

As the child regains control over his movements the therapists must decide if and when standardised objective assessments are to be used. Standardized assessments provide objective findings of the child's performance, based on normative data for the child's age group. It should be stressed that all assessments of the child (both standardized and non-standardized) are of equal importance in realistically assessing the child's functioning within his environment. Standardized tests may give figures indicating the level of the child's ability, but this must be tempered with an awareness of related factors such as fatigue levels, problems with comprehension, cultural factors etc. All assessments should be accompanied with qualitative comments on the child's performance at the time of testing.

Standardized assessments provide readily communicable information (but only to other professionals who are familiar with the test used.) They enable a baseline of ability to be established and to provide an objective framework against which change in the child's abilities over time can be measured.

Test of Visual Perceptual Skills (TVPS) (Gardner 1982)
The purpose of this test is to determine a child's visual – perceptual strengths and weaknesses based on non-motor visual-perceptual testing. It provides norm-based visual perceptual ages for each subtest, visual – perceptual scaled scores for each sub test and visual – perceptual percentiles for each sub – test. By sub-dividing the test into seven discrete areas therapists can pin-point specific areas of deficit and plan a relevant programme of remediation. This test covers the age range 4 to 13 years.

Test of Auditory Perceptual Skills (TAPS) (Gardner 1985)
This test was created to aid examiners in diagnosing children with language

disorders. It is designed to measure six areas of auditory skills of children aged between 4 and 12 years of age. The TAPS provide norms for each subtest in terms of language age, standard scores and percentiles. It is an assessment tool developed to measure a child's functioning in various areas of auditory perception. Any one or a combination of poor performance on the subtest can interefere with a child's reading and/or spelling abilities.

Tests of Visual – Motor Skills – Revised (TVMS-R) (Gardner 1995)
This test measures visual-motor skills in children from 3 years to 13 years 11 months. It is an untimed test of visual-motor skills in which children are requested to copy geometric designs with a pen and paper. Strengths or weaknesses in specific areas are highlighted and can then be used as key starting points for remediation programmes.

Developmental Test of Visual – Motor Integration (VMI) (Beery 1989)
This is a developmental sequence of 24 geometric shapes which have to be copied with a pencil and paper, the primary purpose of the test being to help prevent learning and behavioural problems through early identification. It can be used by children of different cultural backgrounds because geometric shapes are used rather than numbers or letters. It is designed for children aged 3 to 8 years.

Gross Motor Function Measure (Russell et al 1991)
There is still a distinct lack of assessment tools for measuring change in gross motor function in children who have had a head injury. We have used the Gross Motor Function Measure and although it is not specifically validated for children with brain injuries there was a small group of children with head injuries in the original validation data. The test consists of 88 items in 5 dimensions of lying and rolling, sitting, crawling and kneeling, standing, and walking, running and jumping. The level of motor functioning tested is up to a level of ability of a five year old child. The test can take some time to administer (a minimum of 45 minutes) which can be difficult for the child who suffers fatigue. The test can be completed over more than one session as long as it is completed within one week from starting the assessment. Finally, the measure is useful for therapists and parents to choose goal areas for treatment.

The role of the occupational therapist in intermediate rehabilitation

The occupational therapist focuses on the following:

• promoting skills in independent living
• assessing the need for specialised equipment or adaptations to the home or school environment
• developing normal patterns of movement thus facilitating optimum conditions for return of hand function

- assessing and optimising the child's perceptual abilities

Once the child's baseline level of ability has been established, the treatment programme will be designed based on these findings. At this stage the child may have a very limited attention span and may therefore find it difficult to concentrate for any length of time, which will clearly limit the duration of therapy. The occupational therapist's emphasis will be to incorporate therapeutic activities into everday tasks.

Self care skills and orientation

The child will now be actively involved in a programme of rehabilitation, involving periods of therapy, play and rest. It is important for the child to recognise the structure of the day, in order to enhance his orientation.

At this stage parents and child should be provided with daily and weekly timetables, in a form which the child can understand (eg, representational pictures which can be removed, once the child has completed a particular activity). Parents are encouraged to actively involve their child in this process, and to add in names of friends or relatives who may be visiting.

The establishment of a routine and reason to each day is an appropriate motivator for the child to get dressed, washed, eat meals, and carry out all daily life skills. Practising these skills in isolation will provide little motivation for the child, and the practice of such skills at inappropriate times may only serve to reinforce disorientation in time. It is therefore important to carry out such tasks at the appropriate time of day and in the most appropriate location. The use of these well practised activities has further therapeutic benefits. They provide a child with routines based in familiarity, (which give reassurance and maximise the child's opportunity for success), they provide meaningful instances in which parents can be actively involved in their child's rehabilitation throught the day, and provide opportunities for therapeutic advice to be incorporated into normal activities within the child's routine (eg, specific positioning, use of specific communication channels etc). This is important when taking a long-term view of a child who may have residual disabilities, and who will therefore find it helpful to employ an adaptive model of treatment, in which familiar activities may have to be relearnt or carried out in new ways in order to enhance functional abilities.

Promotion of skills in independent living

The strength of the occupational therapist lies in her skills in task analysis (ie breaking down an activity into its component tasks).

For children with visual–spatial difficulties, dressing can be very difficult. It is easiest to encourage the child to participate first in undressing before going to bed or hydrotherapy. Parents are advised to bring in familiar clothing, particularly garments which are not tight fitting. The child should be encouraged to carry out as much of the activity as possible, provided that their movement does not cause further increase in muscle tone by using excessive effort.

For the child with asymmetrical muscle tone (ie hemiplegia) dressing should always be carried out with a stable surface in front of the child, so that clothes can be placed in mid-view and the midline of the child. In order to prevent retraction of the shoulder on the affected side, and in order to promote awareness of this side, the child should always be encouraged to dress this side first. When undressing, the unaffected side should be removed first from garments in order to then assist with removal of garments from the affected side.

Clear, simple verbal or non-verbal assistance should only be given if necessary, with a view to reducing this until it is no longer necessary. Dressing gives a good opportunity to assess the child's ability to sequence a familiar activity correctly and to observe his planning and motor organisational skills. Perceptual skills such as spatial awareness, body awareness, right-left discrimination and figure ground discrimination are all necessary to the process, and the therapist observes the child's ability in all these areas. A child with proprioceptive problems will have difficulty in positioning their joints appropriately and so dressing may be used as a therapeutic medium in which to start to re-establish these normal patterns of movement. For the child with poor skills in recognising objects by texture and shape (eg stereognosis), finding, and being able to fasten buttons without vision will pose great difficulty.

It must be acknowledged that at this stage, the child's information processing skills are likely to be slowed down, even following a mild injury (Giles and Clarke-Wilson 1993) and so repetitive activities will help to reinforce and enhance the child's short and long-term memory skills.

The same process of analysing an acitivty and breaking it down into component tasks can be applied to any activity of daily living (eg eating, drinking, washing) in order establish a programme of therapeutic input.

Assessing the need for specialized equipment or adaptations (home or school)

A child's needs are, understandably, variable. Some children will recover dramatically quickly whilst others will show little recovery. As a general rule, any adaptations are initially temporary and can therefore be modified at the pace of the child's recovery.

Initially, the child may require adapted cutlery or crockery to feel himself, or he may equally need to accommodate a new method of carrying out a task, (getting washed whilst sitting in a chair, rather than standing at the sink). When the child has mobility problems, locomotor, toiletting, bathing and access to his home are issues that need to be addressed. The child may require his home environment to be re-arranged (eg so that he can sleep downstairs initially) or it may be that major building adaptations will need to be initiated, in order to acommodate his major long-term physical needs. At this stage of rehabilitation, contact should be initiated with the child's local community services, and in particular with the local social services occupational therapist who will be responsible for jointly assessing, and then providing, specific equipment/adaptations.

Facilitation of optimum conditions for return of hand function

Close liaison and working jointly with the physiotherapist, the occupational therapist works to facilitiate the child's recovery of bimanual hand function. If increased or fluctuating tone is present, preparatory work should first be carried out to normalize tone, in order to maximise the child's success at carrying out a fine motor activity. This work should not be embarked upon until sufficient muscle control is achieved in the child's trunk, head, shoulders and arms. Intricate activity may cause an increase of muscle tone if an activity is too effortful. If the muscle tone is high the initial movements in the hands should be relaxed, smooth, and only as gross movements. Initially, this may take the form of 'batting' movements away from the body, interspersed with weight-bearing or extension of the affected upper limb in order to inhibit the effects of spasticity. Bimanual function is aimed for by involving the child in activities or games requiring two hands. To incorporate inhibition of tone the child may be encouraged to use his affected side as his 'assistant' hand. Initially such function may simply require the child to stabilise a toy using two hands, with arms in extension. Grasping of objects precludes releasing them, but again, this must be asked of the child if the act of grasping increases flexor tone in the upper limbs and trunk. Once the child has the possibility of active finger extension then the release of objects into more precisely defined areas should follow in order to improve accuracy of placing.

The choice of activities used is influenced by the child's age, culture, memory, attention span, hobbies and interests. The therapist's skill at creating optimum conditions for specific therapeutic benefits are greatly challenged. Ideally, the child should find the sessions motivating and fun, in order to gain his maximum co-operation over what can be long periods of rehabilitation. A wide variety of tasks, both novel and familiar can be presented in ways which invite the child to explore further.

In addition to physical recovery, recovery of sensation is very important to the child's awareness of movement. Proprioceptive feedback about joint and muscle position, temperature and pain, and tactile receptors all provide the child with vital information prior to planning movements, and may be impaired following head injury. For this reason, the importance of the child feeling the sensation of normal movement cannot be over stressed. A child learns about movement through the sensation of feeling it. It is therefore crucial that the child does not learn poor quality movements which may later impede optimal physical recovery.

When the child is able to maintain as normal a postural tone as possible, activities are provided to encourage forearm pronation and supination and wrist extension. Opposition of the thumb to all fingers is desirable for return of functional grip (which will be necessary for writing and carrying out all tasks requiring dexterity). Activities to refine flow, control and speed are designed to facilitate return of the child's previous skills. However, if this can only be partially achieved, the occupational therapist will assess the need for adaptations to the way in which the child records school work. For the senior school age child the therapist may introduce keyboard skills to the treatment programme and expand this to the use of a world processor in school. The child who has such physical difficulty in recording work with pen and paper, but who demonstrates proficiency with a word processor is a candidate for a 'Statement of Special Educational Need'. This is a legal document, reviewed annually, outlining specific provisions which are needed for the child in class. Through this process, recommendations such as access to a word processor, or extra time for examinations can be arranged. This is discussed in more detail in Chapters 8 and 10.

Assessing and maximizing the child's perceptual abilities

The occupational therapist utilises a combination of familiar and unfamiliar situations in which to assess and treat the child's skills. Qualitative assessments are first made in realistic settings in order to give the child optimal cues from familiarity. In later stages, when the child is in a more alert state, and away from the busy ward environment, the therapist may employ objective standardised tests such as the Test of Visual Perceptual Skills (Gardner) in order to provide a baseline.

LATER REHABILITATION

This stage of progress is taken to coincide with the time the child starts the hospital school. It is likely that at this time the child is still a hospital in-patient, but, almost certainly, rehabilitation will continue following discharge. The local Education authority usually (but not invariably) will provide transport for local children who attend the hospital school.

As with early rehabilitation, the frequency of physiotherapy, hydrotherapy and occupational therapy sessions which are required once a child is recovering from a brain injury still has to be objectively tested (Campbell 1991). Obviously, the physiotherapy input will decline as physical progress occurs and when there is a change of priorities for the child, particularly as the educational/cognitive rehabilitation (and input) assumes greater importance.

Most physical recovery following head and other brain injuries occurs during the first year, and this has also been our clinical experience (Scott-Jupp *et al.* 1992). This often leads the physiotherapist to feel a sense of needing to maximize the child's spontaneous recovery and physical potential at a time when he has the opportunity to receive daily therapy, a situation which may not be possible once the child has been transferred to local therapy services in view of the ever-increasing workloads (and often limited availability) of community physiotherapy staff. As with treatment in the early stages, a balance needs to be achieved between the treatment ideal and the child's overall needs.

Goal-setting

The use of goal setting as part of therapy treatment programmes for children with neurological impairment has been shown to aid motor progress (Bower *et al.* 1996). As for children with cerebral palsy, the goals selected for brain-injured children need to be functional and achievable, hence they need to take into consideration the child's stage of physical recovery as well as the likely potential for further recovery. If parents are involved in this process it can sometimes help their acceptance of a child's long-term disability.

Treatment

The aims and principles of treatment are identical to those described earlier in this chapter. The specific positions used for treatment, as well as treatment techniques, will continue to be adapted to meet each child's individual needs and take into consideration his physical and additional problems. At this stage the child may be a little more tolerant of treatment and to changes of position; he may also fatigue less easily than in the early stages.

Most treatment sessions are usually carried out in the relevant therapy department rather than in the school classroom. However, treatment may often be followed up with functional positioning in the classroom; for example, for a child who cannot stand unaided, a period of standing in a standing frame in class may be appropriate after a treatment session. As with earlier stages, if physiotherapy treatment is to be effective, physical management needs to be continued throughout the day and incorporated into the daily routines of ward, school, and home. If it is appropriate, the family are asked to carry out specific activities, and treatment goals are negotiated with them, so making treatment as relevant as possible to the home situation.

Physical management in the classroom

The physiotherapist and occupational therapist are in regular contact with teaching staff in order to discuss the child's physical abilities (and difficulties) and, whenever appropriate, advice will include suggestions for a daily therapy programme, updated on a regular basis, which can be undertaken in the classroom. This may be carried out by suitably trained classroom assistants.

The general philosophy of physical treatment is to encourage the child's use of as normal a movement as possible, without excessive effort and avoiding causing an increase in muscle tone. This emphasizes the need to pitch the child's physical activities at an appropriate level for their physical capabilities, with teaching and care staff giving assistance when required. This helps to avoid unnecessary frustration for the child and allows him to achieve part of the activity and to relearn motor control. Praise is given for 'correct' movements. Practical issues, such as whether or not the child is allowed to walk, are discussed and reviewed regularly.

Environment and equipment

Advice in this area obviously overlaps and combines with advice from other members of the team, particularly the occupational therapist. The child's sitting position in the classroom in terms of appropriate (including special) seating, appropriate desk or table height, as well as using tables of the right size and incline, together with the need to present work and the teaching materials in the correct way, are all important factors.

The layout of the classroom and the need to accommodate special equipment, allowing wheelchair access, and manoeuvrability both in and around the classroom is discussed, as is the use of standing frames and the needs of children who walk with mobility aids.

Joint working

Throughout this stage of rehabilitation there will always be the need for continual assessment and review of each child's difficulties and for all treatment to be planned to meet individual requirements, taking into consideration the overall medical and physical condition as well as the additional demands of school. Wherever possible, treatment should still incorporate materials which the child was familiar with before the injury, e.g. cassettes, footballs, dolls, etc. This requires continued involvement and contact with the family, even though they are not usually present for as many treatment sessions as they were in the earlier stages of rehabilitation. Knowledge of each child's cognitive deficits as well as their problems in attention, concentration, and behaviour, together with details of their pre-morbid status, continue to be essential to allow the therapist to plan effective therapy sessions and to make treatment as relevant and age-appropriate as is practicable. There is obviously an ongoing need to maintain multidisciplinary assessment of the child's progress (BPA 1991) as well as discussion of appropriate management techniques. One mechanism for this is through the the Team's weekly head-injury meetings.

A further means of joint working are joint-treatment sessions. In the early stages of rehabilitation this commonly involves therapists, nursing staff, and play specialists; in the later stages joint physiotherapy and occupational therapy or speech therapy sessions assume more importance and relevance. However, joint sessions can involve any of the team-members including, when appropriate, parents and carers.

Continued liaison between therapists and the school staff is essential in order to coordinate therapy appointments with the child's school curriculum; this occurs when the therapists and link teacher for the team have their weekly planning meeting. The therapists and other team-members are involved in regular school reviews for the child whilst he continues to attend the hospital school.

Preparation for discharge from hospital therapies and liaison with local (including community) therapists

The timing of, and preparation for, discharge to local services is a team decision and planning discharge requires many factors to be considered. Liaison with the child's local services is essential not only to ensure continuity of treatment and to minimize any unnecessary delay but also to help prepare the child and his family for discharge and a change of services. From the therapists viewpoint this involves:

- initial telephone contact with the local physiotherapist and occupational therapist
- meeting the therapists with the parents in a joint visit at Alder Hey, or possibly visiting the new school with the child to meet the therapy staff there
- keeping the parents informed about liaison between the different therapists.

It is important to remember that the child and family are likely to have had a great deal of contact with members of the team at a very traumatic and emotional time; hence they often make quite close relationships and the change to new services is likely to be difficult. This change often coincides with the time when a child's persisting disability is becoming evident to the family and therefore considerable support and discussion needs to be provided.

Spatial-awareness difficulties take on a new significance when the child is able to go home. He may have problems judging speed and distance, which makes crossing the road potentially hazardous. The child will often stand for a long time making sure that there is no traffic, by which time another car has inevitably appeared; this is, in fact, more common than crossing the road too quickly. The dangers of traffic should be strongly emphasized and if there is any doubt about the child's level of competence he should not be allowed to cross on his own. The child may need to reorientate himself to his local area or school. Changing classes can also be a particularly stressful situation when the child has to negotiate crowded corridors and stairs, remember the correct books, where the next classroom is located, and when the next lesson is to start.

Whilst the role of the educational psychologist is to assess cognitive skills in relation to educational needs, the role of the occupational therapist is to assess and relate cognitive abilities to function. It is clearly important that knowledge learned in a new situation is able to be generalized into other situations. Work focuses particularly on short-term memory and spatial awareness skills; this includes a number of functional memory tasks, including remembering where articles have been left and ensuring that they are returned to the same place. The family are encouraged to take some responsibility for similar tasks at home. A diary is often used to facilitate this task; if short-term memory continues to be a significant problem, additional strategies will be required – often using wall-charts and noticeboards to highlight events and activities that are not to be missed. More detailed discussion can be found in Chapter 8.

MANAGEMENT OF THE CHILD WHO FAILS TO PROGRESS

Unfortunately, not all children will make a good recovery after a brain injury. Children with a long-term severe neurological deficit will need careful management to minimize the effects of altered postural tone and loss of normal movement, which may cause contractures and deformities. Correct positioning is vital in the management of these children. Specialist equipment will be important in helping to provide alternative positions, including a standing frame, static chair, or sidelying frame which may be used at school, home or, if possible, both (particularly during school holidays).

Assessment of the child's seating needs will be required in order to provide him with an appropriate wheelchair or buggy. This can be organized through the local wheelchair service. If the child lives outside the catchment area of the hospital, the wheelchair service can organize funding from the child's local district – although this is not always straightforward!

A great deal of planning is required if and when these children are to return home. Close links will need to be set up with community therapists to ensure that the home is suitably prepared and any equipment that is needed is at least ordered, if not already available within the home. Older children who require assistance with lifting may need to be supplied with a hoist and/or stair lift. It is obviously very important that the parents are confident and proficient in handling these children, as they will have complex long-term needs, which can be a heavy burden (both physically and emotionally) to parents. Prior to the child's discharge, treatment sessions should concentrate on basic management issues with the parents, including carrying and handling the child and addressing all aspects of daily living.

Where a child does not achieve full recovery the educational psychologist will identify the difficulties and be involved in securing an appropriate school placement. Where possible the school or community therapist will visit the hospital (or specific therapy department) to ensure a smooth transfer. This will involve liaision regarding the child's assessment and treatment programme and current level of functioning. Occasional problems occur when local authorities are not able to provide the therapy programme that the child has been receiving in the hospital because of inadequate, or lack of, staff and resources. The early and judicious involvement of the legal profession (including the courts) may be useful in these situations by securing early or interim financial support (eg, through compensation or 'damages') which could facilitate the provision of some therapy sessions, costly special equipment (eg, communication aids) or home adaptations.

The occupational therapist will liaise with the local authority occupational therapist if adaptations and structural alterations are required, usually as soon as these needs are identified and certainly well before the child is discharged from the hospital ward. Specialized equipment may be needed, such as an adapted chair or bath seat, and again such needs are passed on to the community occupational therapist as soon as possible, as it may take many days if not weeks to provide this equipment within the home. One or more joint home visits are frequently arranged in order to ensure a smooth transition from hospital to home, which is an essential component of a child's rehabilitation – both physically and emotionally. This transfer of care – from the hospital to the community – is also very important for the family. They may have come to rely heavily upon the well-resourced and well-established hospital-based services, and if the necessary equipment and ongoing therapy and support is not made available within the home and community at the time of transfer, this may have significant adverse effects on their own physical and emotional rehabilitation and recovery.

The therapists continue to work closely with the family to ensure that they are able to, and do, carry out the therapy programmes at home. Following discharge, the families, children, and local professionals are encouraged to maintain contact with the hosptial rehabilitation team for advice, and, when necessary, support. The local authority occupational therapists may provide a long-term service, upgrading equipment as the child grows or his needs change. It is hoped that hospitalization should represent only a small part of the child's life that he has coped with, and adapted to, before being fully integrated back into his family and school life.

REFERENCES

Beery, K.E. (1989). *The Developmental Test of Visual-Motor Integration*. Modern Curriculum Press, Toronto.

Bobath, K. and Bobath, B. (1984). Management of motor disorders of children with cerebral palsy. In *Clinics in Developmental Medicine*, no. **90**, (ed. D. Scrutton), pp. 6-18.

Bower, E., McLellan, D.L., Arney, J., and Campbell, M.J. (1996). A randomized controlled trial of different intensities of physiotherapy and different goal-setting procedures in 44 children with cerebral palsy. *Developmental Medicine and Child Neurology*, **38**, 226–38

British Paediatric Association (BPA) and British Association of Paediatric Surgeons Joint Standing Committee on Childhood Accidents. (1991). *Report of a Working Party: Guidelines on the management of head injuries in childhood*. BPA, London.

Bryce, J. (1972). Facilitation of movement – Bobath approach. *Physiotherapy*, **58**, 403–7.

Bryce, J. (1976). The management of spasticity in children. *Physiotherapy*, **62**, 353–7.

Burns, Y. and Paratz, P. (1993). The effect of respiratory physiotherapy on intracranial pressure, mean arterial pressure, cerebral perfusion pressure and end tidal carbon dioxide in ventilated neurosurgical patients. *Physiotherapy Theory and Practice*, **9**, 3–11.

Campbell, S. (1991). *Paediatric neurologic physical therapy* (2nd edn). , Churchill Livingstone, London, New York.

Gardner, M.F. (1982). *Test of Visual-Perceptual Skills (non-motor)*. Psychological and Educational Publications Inc., California.

Gardner, M.F. (1985). *Test of Auditory-Perceptual Skills*. Psychological and Educational Publications Inc., California.

Gardner, M.F. (1995). *Test of Visual-Motor Skills – Revised*. Psychological and Educational Publications Inc., California.

Giles, G. M. and Clarke-Wilson, J. (1993). Brain injury rehabilitation: a neurofunctional approach. *Therapy in Practice*, **no. 33**, Chapman and Hall, London.

Hall, D. M. B., Johnson, S. L. J., and Middleton, J. (1990). Rehabilitation of head injured children. *Archives of Disease in Childhood*, **65**, 553–6.

Henderson, S.E., and Sugden, D.A. (1992). Movement Assessment Battery for Children. The Psychological Corporation, New York.

Kidd, G., Lawes, N., and Musa, I. (1992). *Understanding neuromuscular plasticity – a basis for clinical rehabilitation*. Edward Arnold, London.

Le Roux, A.A. (1993). Teler: the concept. *Physiotherapy*, **79**, 755–8

Lynch, M. and Grisogono, V. (1991). *Strokes and head injuries – a guide for patients, families, friends, and carers*, p.116. John Murray, London.

Scott-Jupp, R., Marlow, N., Seddon, N., and Rosenbloom, L. (1992). Rehabilitation and outcome after severe head injury. *Archives of Disease in Childhood*, **67**, 222–6.

Martin, K. (1983). Therapeutic pool activities for young children in a community facility. In *Aquatics: a revived approach to paediatric management* (ed. F. Dulcy), p.66 The Howarth Press, London.

Russell, D. J., Rosenbaum, P. L., Cadman, D. T., Gowland, C., Hardy, S., and Jarvis, S. (1989). The gross motor function measure: a means to evaluate the effects of physical therapy. *Developmental Medicine and Child Neurology*, **31**, 341–52.

6

Managing feeding and swallowing problems in the brain-injured child

Siobhan McMahon

INTRODUCTION

The child with a severe brain injury who has required ventilatory support will have been nourished by enteral or parenteral (intravenous) feeding. For the minority of children who have to remain on the intensive care unit for some time and require prolonged intravenous feeding, their metabolic response and nutritional status are crucial: this is clearly an important issue but falls outside the remit of this chapter, and is well reviewed by Roberts (1995). Fortunately the vast majority of children with brain injuries do not require long-term ventilatory support, intensive care, or prolonged intravenous ('total parenteral') nutrition. As the child is weaned from the ventilator and begins to show signs of arousal, the reintroduction of oral feeding is often viewed as the next important step in the child's recovery.

However, the child's ability to eat and drink can not be managed in isolation. Any problems he has will reflect not only specific problems with swallowing but also his emotional, physical, and communication difficulties.

The child may have only fleeting periods of wakefulness and alertness. It is important that decisions regarding the reintroduction of oral feeding are influenced by the child's readiness, and not by the understandable wishes of the child's parents, or others caring for him, to 'progress'.

The child must be carefully and thoroughly assessed before he or his parents are encouraged to commence oral feeding. It is important for the child and his family to see positive signs of recovery, and therefore professionals involved in the child's care need to ensure, as far as possible, that he is not allowed to start something, such as eating, which then has to be stopped when found to be inappropriate. Careful liaison between all members of the team caring for the child, particularly the medical and nursing staff, is therefore crucial.

The child's family should receive a simple explanation of the issues involved in the reintroduction of oral feeding and withdrawal of tube feeding, i.e. ensuring that the child can swallow safely and can meet his nutritional needs without additional support. The family and, where appropriate, the child should be prepared for the procedures involved in assessing his ability to swallow safely, but should also be aware that this is only one element in the process of the rehabilitation of oral feeding. They should also know that it is likely to be a gradual process, occurring over at least a few or several days rather than by a sudden, complete withdrawal of tube feeding.

Parents also need to be helped to understand that all aspects of the child's neurological impairment will have some effect on his ability to feed and swallow. For example, it may be difficult for the child to tolerate an appropriate sitting position, even with the aid of adapted seating. His poor head and trunk control will affect his ability to maintain his head and neck in a suitable and safe position for eating and drinking and difficulty with fine motor skills leaves the child entirely dependent and unable to feed himself. In addition, he may have very limited means of communication and therefore be unable to express basic needs such as hunger and thirst; he cannot influence the type of food he is given, when he receives it and at what rate, or express any specific preferences he may have.

ASSESSING THE CHILD'S ABILITY TO SWALLOW

Before the child can be allowed to commence oral feeding, his ability to swallow safely must be established.

Swallowing is a highly complex motor act, requiring fine control and coordination of breathing and swallowing. If this coordination is impaired, the child may breath material into the lungs, which is known as aspiration and can lead to chest infection, pneumonia, and long-term damage to the lungs. Aspiration may also exacerbate any pre-existing asthma, and both this and pneumonia may necessitate a return to the intensive care unit and even ventilatory support, with an obvious (and potentially prolonged) delay in the child's overall rehabilitation programme.

Children who have sustained neurological damage are at significant risk of aspiration due to impairment of the swallow reflex and reduced or ineffective cough reflexes. They are therefore prone to the potentially serious consequences of aspiration and these risks are heightened in the child who is immobile and may already have had respiratory problems associated with any other injuries (eg: fractured ribs).

A proportion of neurologically impaired patients who aspirate do so silently, i.e. without outward signs such as coughing. Conversely, some children who do cough during swallowing are able to protect their airway by the cough and do not actually aspirate.

While the child's alertness and physical and oral-motor skills can be assessed through observation and during 'trial' swallows of carefully selected material, the use of the X-ray technique known as videofluroscopy, as described by

Griggs *et al.* (1989), is now widely accepted as the gold-standard method of assessing swallowing and demonstrating aspiration.

VIDEOFLUROSCOPY

Videofluroscopy involves taking a moving X-ray image of the child attempting to swallow material of various consistencies. As normal swallowing occurs rapidly, the X-ray images are recorded on videotape for later analysis and also to provide a baseline for future studies. Close cooperation between the radiologist and the speech and language therapist is required to ensure that useful information about the child's ability to swallow fluids, semi-solid, and solid material is obtained with minimum exposure to radiation. The aim is for the examination to replicate normal feeding as far as possible, so careful attention must be paid to appropriate positioning of the child, with help from the physiotherapist (or occupational therapist) where necessary. In addition, a parent or other familiar adult is asked to feed the child and familiar foods and his normal utensils are used whenever possible.

The videofluroscopy examination enables a careful assessment of the child's ability to swallow to be carried out. Any aspiration can be demonstrated, and the effect of altering factors such as the consistency of the food or the position in which the child is fed, can be evaluated. For example, aspiration may occur because of a delay in the triggering of a swallow reflex. Thus material is held in the pharynx for far longer than normal and as the child breathes it is aspirated into the airway. If the child does not have a protective cough reflex, this material may enter the lungs, causing respiratory problems.

Just as the child's swallow reflex may be delayed, he may also have a delayed cough reflex which is triggered after the material has passed the larynx, and thus does not protect him from the consequences of aspiration. It is therefore important to make the child's parents, and others caring for him, aware of the fact that although the child has been heard to cough, this does not necessarily indicate that he has an adequate protective cough reflex.

Videofluroscopy therefore provides an objective measure of the child's ability to swallow safely. Clearly, the child who aspirates all the types of food tested will remain unsafe for oral feeding and require a further period of tube feeding before his ability to swallow is reassessed. However sometimes the child with a slightly delayed swallow reflex can be observed to safely swallow material of a smooth, semi-solid consistency, such as a rusk or thick custard, although aspiration of both fluids and thickened liquids may be observed. This child could be carefully reintroduced to some oral feeding, with a selected diet of suitable foods, while continuing to have fluids given via a nasogastric tube.

REINTRODUCTION OF EATING AND DRINKING

Once objective assessment has indicated that the child is able to swallow safely, the gradual reintroduction of oral feeding can begin. As described above, some children will require a restricted diet in order to prevent aspiration, which may involve continued use of a nasogastric tube or, in others, the addition of thickening agents to the child's fluids if videofluroscopic studies have indicated that this is safe.

In addition, some children will continue to require nutritional support because they cannot manage to consume an adequate volume of food in a reasonable time. This may be due to the child's reduced alertness, fatiguability, or significant oral-motor difficulties. Rehabilitation of oral feeding should proceed gradually at a pace which is comfortable for the child; the temptation to withdraw nutritional support as soon as a safe reflex swallow has been demonstrated should be avoided.

In common with children with developmental feeding difficulties, attention must be paid to all the factors which may influence the child's ability to eat and drink as independently as possible.

Environmental factors

Particularly in the early stages of recovery, the brain-injured child may find concentrating and attending to a single task difficult, and therefore it is helpful to reduce unnecessary distractions and background noise. The child needs to be encouraged to concentrate on eating and drinking and should not be expected to carry out other activities, such as watching television or talking about an unrelated topic, simultaneously.

While the child may eventually benefit from socializing with others at mealtimes, this needs to be introduced carefully and sensitively, especially in the child who is aware of his physical limitations and who may be embarrassed by spillage, drooling, etc.

Positioning

Appropriate supportive seating and careful positioning is essential to enable the child to eat and/or drink as safely and as independently as possible. Close liaison with the physiotherapist is required as the child will require careful and thorough assessment to determine the optimum position for him during mealtimes. It is important to ensure that both the child's parents and the ward staff are aware of his particular positioning and seating needs.

Communication

The brain-injured child with feeding difficulties is also likely to have significant impairment of his communication skills. This means he may be unable to clearly indicate when he is hungry or thirsty, what he would like to eat, what he likes or dislikes, etc. It is important that the child is given some opportunity to choose what he would like to eat, both to maintain his interest in eating and, as described elsewhere, to promote his ability to communicate in a realistic, meaningful situation. This can be encouraged through the use of pointing or simple communication charts as soon as the child is able to manage this.

In addition to allowing him some control over the type of foods he is offered, it is important that the child who is unable to feed independently is encouraged to indicate when he is ready for the next mouthful, when he would like a drink, etc. so that he is able to take as active a part as possible in the management of his difficulties.

Taste and texture

In the early stages of recovery, eating and drinking may be difficult and effortful for the child; therefore it is important to ensure that the foods he is offered are visually attractive and tasty, to develop his motivation and maintain his interest in eating. This is particularly important where the child can only manage a limited range of food textures, as puréed and mashed foods can look particularly unappetizing if not carefully prepared and presented. Maintaining variety is also important to prevent the child becoming bored and disinterested.

The child who has oral motor difficulties, making it difficult for him to manipulate food in the mouth and chew, will need a carefully graded programme for the reintroduction of foods of increasingly difficult textures. Some children will also require help to maintain jaw control and/or lip closure during eating and drinking. Specific management strategies for particular difficulties are beyond the scope of this chapter but are well described elsewhere – see Arvedson (1993).

Utensils

The selection of utensils which are appropriate for, and acceptable to, the child should be undertaken in close conjunction with the occupational therapists. A wide variety of adapted cutlery and cups are available and should be selected to meet the child's individual needs, promoting safe-feeding practice (for example, avoiding the use of metal cutlery in the child who has a bite reflex and is in danger of breaking teeth), independence (for example, providing a large bore handle so that the child can use a spoon independently), and encouraging the development of better oral motor control (for example, using straw-drinking to promote lip rounding).

As with all other aspects of his rehabilitation, the child with feeding and swallowing difficulties resulting from both traumatic and non-traumatic brain injury requires careful assessment and a well-coordinated, multidisciplinary approach to his management to ensure that he receives the consistent care required to enable him to regain as much independence as possible.

Children with more severe brain injuries frequently develop additional gastrointestinal difficulties, including gastro-oesophageal reflux, gastritis, and general (and often severe) dysmotility of the entire small and large intestines, often resulting in painful colic and constipation. Whilst a number of these symptoms may be amenable to different medical therapies, it is not uncommon for some of these children to require surgical intervention, including fundoplication (to reduce or prevent gastro-oesophageal reflux) and a feeding gastrostomy. During and throughout the rehabilitation programme, the speech and language therapist remains a key member of the team in planning the most appropriate method of feeding the child and contributing to these medical/surgical decisions.

REFERENCES

Arvedson, J. (1993). Management of swallowing problems. in *Pediatric swallowing and feeding* (ed. J. Arvedson and L. Brodsky). Whurr Publishers, London.
Griggs, C. A., Jones, P. M., and Lee, R. F. (1989) Videofluroscopic investigations of feeding disorders of children with multiple handicap. *Developmental Medicine and Child Neurology*, **31**, 303–8.
Roberts, P.R. (1995). Nutrition in the head-injured patient. *New Horizons*, **3**, 506–17.

7

Speech and language difficulties

Siobhan McMahon

INTRODUCTION

Speech and language therapists have an important role to play as members of the multidisciplinary team caring for the brain-injured child. While many children can and do make excellent recoveries from traumatic brain injury, most will require some help with communication, even if this is just for a short time. In addition there is increasing evidence that many children with brain injuries go on to have long-term difficulties with some aspect of communication. Unfortunately, there is very little information available on the nature and treatment of communication impairment following severe brain injury in childhood, and therapists therefore have to rely on knowledge derived from other communication-impaired populations to both inform and guide their management of these children.

Many different professional groups are involved in the rehabilitation of children with brain injuries and their management needs to be carefully coordinated to ensure that each child receives consistent care.

EARLY MANAGEMENT

Traumatic brain injury can cause a variety of disorders of communication, affecting the child's ability to understand and/or use language. Once the child begins to show some signs of awareness, early management should focus on meeting his immediate communicative needs in a functional manner. Early intervention aims to help the child to communicate however he can, and not necessarily to teach specific skills or address particular areas of deficit. It should also help parents and others involved in the child's care to see how he can communicate, and how they can reinforce and extend any residual skills the child has. The child needs to be helped and encouraged to use his own strategies for communication. In the very early stages the child is likely to use only simple strategies, such as crying when distressed, but it is important that adults respond to these rather than trying to teach the child *new* ways of communicating. For example, strategies such as 'blink once for "yes" and twice for "no"' result only in disappointment when the child does not use them. Such strategies also take the focus away from observing and responding appropriately to any communicative behaviours the child already has, leading parents and carers to try and teach specific behaviours which *they* feel would be helpful.

Parents need to be made aware that a child in the early stages of recovery is not in a good position to learn new strategies for communication and therefore the adults need to focus their attention on interpreting any communicative behaviours the child is using. For example, parents can be encouraged to notice and describe what the child does when he is upset, what he does when he hears something familiar or strange, comforting or frightening, etc. This helps them to become aware of their child's responses to a range of stimuli, even where these are limited. It also helps parents from an early stage to take an active part in their child's treatment, rather than feeling frustrated that they have failed to get him to blink or nod his head appropriately.

Because early intervention should be based on what the child *can* rather than cannot do, if he does appear to have some understanding he can be encouraged to demonstrate *how* he can communicate. For example, questions such as 'Show me what you can do when you mean "yes'" help the child to develop communication strategies which he understands, has the physical skills to produce, and is therefore likely to use. This is a more child oriented approach than giving instructions such as blink/ nod your head/ wriggle your toes if you mean 'yes"' etc. and helps the child to remain in some control over his own communication skills. More typically, however the child will show only fleeting awareness of his environment, and his communication difficulties will result primarily from his lack of understanding rather than his inability to speak.

As the child begins to show some signs of recovery, his first communicative behaviours are likely to be in response to unpleasant stimuli, including pain or discomfort as these often provoke strong reactions. It is important that these initial responses are seen as a sign of progress, as the child is beginning to respond to his environment. Parents can be helped to feel that they are assisting their child to recover by providing a familiar and reassuring presence, and they should be encouraged to help their child now, rather than spending their time constantly trying to observe, or work towards a distant goal.

Parents' existing knowledge of their own child and his likes, dislikes, interests and hobbies provides essential information for the therapist working with the child, enabling input to be tailored specifically to the child's interests. It is also a useful means of encouraging parents to continue to see themselves as 'experts' in their own child's care and rehabilitation, rather than becoming the recipients of 'expert' help from the professionals currently caring for their child.

Very early intervention therefore concentrates on helping parents and carers to see, understand and reinforce any communicative behaviour the child has, however limited this may be. Communicative behaviours can include sounds and movements the child makes when he is uncomfortable, wants changing, is hungry or thirsty, etc. The responsibility is therefore placed on the parents and carers to observe and understand the child's behaviours, rather than on the child to develop new communication skills at the time when he is least well-equipped to do so.

Any early intervention should focus on meeting the child's immediate needs, which will depend on his level of awareness and the severity of his injury. The majority of children with severe injuries will have some impairment of their ability to understand spoken language. While the child's lack of speech may be the most obvious problem, impairments of receptive language (understanding) should not be overlooked and must be managed appropriately.

Modification of the environment

The brain-injured child in the early stages of recovery is likely to have difficulty making sense of the hospital environment. He is in an unfamiliar place surrounded by strangers, and may have impaired vision, hearing, and understanding. He may be unaware of events leading up to his admission and the combination of these factors result in a frightened and confused child.

In the early stages of recovery the child may have great difficulty attending to specific stimuli. For example, he may be unable to separate foreground from background noise so has difficulty understanding speech when there is extraneous noise from items such as televisions, radios, and computer games.

Hospital wards are busy, noisy places which can be extremely frightening to the child who cannot understand much of what is going on around him. Reduction of background noise, such as televisions and radios, can help the child focus his attention onto his current activity and may make it easier for him to understand simple language. Similarly, preventing several people from speaking at once and simplifying the language used in terms of both sentence structure and vocabulary can also be helpful in enabling the child to understand.

As with other groups of language-impaired children, using plenty of repetition and restricting topics of conversation to the present are important factors in promoting understanding of spoken language. Parents and others caring for the child can be encouraged to use short, simple phrases, relating their language to everyday activities focused on the child's care and activities. As the child begins to show signs of improvement, conversational topics can be expanded using concrete materials such as familiar toys and story books or photographs of events such as family holidays, Christmas, and birthday parties.

It is important to ensure that the whole team, including the child's parents understands the importance of not bombarding or overloading the child with language which is too complex as this encourages the child to ignore spoken language and rely on environmental cues to make some sense of what is going on around him.

Intervention for the child with profound impairment

Many children will move through the stage of reduced awareness and limited responses in a few days or weeks. However, a small number of children will remain profoundly impaired, with little sign of change or improvement. For these children, intervention must include visual, auditory, and tactile stimulation, with the emphasis on describing the child's communicative behaviours in response to stimulation.

Emphasis should also be placed on consistent management at home and school and specific approaches designed for other children with profound and multiple disabilities, such as the profiling of early communication skills (Kiernan and Reid 1987) and the use of objects of reference, are equally appropriate for children with severe brain injury making minimal progress.

Aided communication

In the early stages of recovery the aim is to provide the child with a means of expressing his basic needs, e.g. pain, hunger, and toileting needs, as soon as he is aware enough to do so. As the child becomes more alert and responsive he can begin to make use of methods of initiating communication. He may be able to vocalize or to activate some type of buzzer to get attention and then respond to simple yes/no questions such as 'Do you want a drink?' or to indicate his needs by selecting pictures on a simple symbol board.

The term 'alternative and augmentative communication' (AAC) is used to describe any system used to enable an individual with impaired speech and language skills to communicate. Communication may be through gestures, signs, symbols or use of an electronic communication aid. In the early stages of recovery, the use of a simple communication chart (see Fig. 7.1) may help to reduce the frustration of the child and those caring for him. Simple communication charts, giving the child the opportunity to express his everyday needs, can easily be made using readily available materials. Several commercial symbol packages are now available (e.g. Boardmaker by Mayer-Johnson), but the basic requirements are that the communication chart is custom-made to reflect the child's individual needs, that the symbols are clear and unambiguous, and that the child can use it easily. Obviously, consideration must therefore be given to the child's visual abilities, his cognitive skills in interpreting the symbols, his physical ability to indicate the appropriate item, and his intention and motivation to communicate. The choice of symbols is also important; they should enable the child to communicate his basic needs, such as making requests and expressing simple emotions.

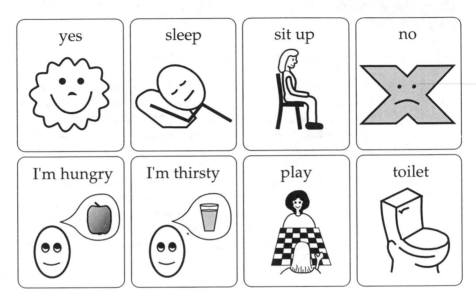

Fig. 7.1 Simple communication chart

Electronic communication aids, which can be programmed to 'speak' a range of phrases at the touch of a key or switch, can be particularly useful as the voice output is usually more motivating for the child than merely indicating symbols on a chart. A wide variety of communication aids are now available which use digitized speech so the voice of a familiar person can be recorded and used. Switching systems allow even children with very poor and limited physical abilities to access this type of equipment, and for the more able child with reading and spelling skills, aids which 'speak' a message typed on a keyboard can be useful.

A variety of communication aids can therefore be used to maximize the child's ability to communicate in the early stages of his recovery. Whilst some children may require this form of communication support in the long term, for many it will be a short-term strategy to provide the child with adequate functional communication. For further information about aided communication see *Communication aids and access to computer technology* (Barrett and Herriotts 1995).

In order to learn to use any type of AAC system the child must be provided with meaningful opportunities to communicate. It is too easy for children, particularly when in a strange environment and with significantly impaired abilities, to become very passive and unresponsive. Thus the child must be given every opportunity to express choices and to have some control over his environment in order to maintain his motivation to communicate and develop his skills to do so.

Promoting Functional Communication Skills

The child's communication skills, however limited, must therefore be used throughout the day in a way which clearly influences what happens to him. Thus the child should be given the chance to choose what he wants to wear, play with, eat, etc. even though, particularly in the early stages of recovery, it may not be clear whether or not he is able to make active choices. For example, the child could be shown two tapes, the adult then waiting for the child to indicate which one he wants played by looking at or reaching towards it. Where the child is not *clearly* able to do this, then prompting the desired response and also providing the opportunity for the child to choose on a regular basis promotes the development of this skill.

As the child's ability to communicate is severely impaired, the adults in his environment need to use every available opportunity to encourage the child to use his residual skills. Where the child is using 'yes' or 'no' responses, which can utilize any movement the child can reliably achieve, but will most usually be a nod or shake of the head, thumbs up or down, etc., then the responsibility for ensuring that the questions can be answered by 'yes' or 'no' must rest firmly with the adult, i.e. 'Are you thirsty?' not 'Do you want blackcurrant or orange juice?'. It is also important to remember at this stage that communication requires effort and may be quite arduous for the child so he should only be asked questions which help to influence his care or environment – and not just to practise 'yes' and 'no' signals. Where the child does need to practise making clear signals then this should be incorporated into a playful activity where the use of the signal becomes meaningful for the child, rather than expecting the child to respond to a series of pointless questions.

Expression of choice needs to be incorporated into virtually all of the child's day-to-day activities, such as dressing and self-help, e.g. choosing items of clothing, where to sit at a table, TV programmes, things to do, etc. Providing the child with this opportunity to express himself is crucial in maintaining his motivation to communicate, particularly as he becomes more alert and increasingly aware of his difficulties.

As the child improves, situations can be carefully engineered to encourage the reluctant child to use his communication skills, although this must be done carefully to ensure he is not unduly frustrated. For example, if the child drops something or has difficulty fastening buttons the adult can wait and see if he asks for help rather than automatically 'helping' as soon as the problem arises. Similarly, the adult can 'forget' to give the child an item essential for a particular activity, such as a fork or pen, and wait for the child to indicate this. In this way, everyday events can be used to give the child opportunities to develop and practise useful skills in a realistic situation.

The brain injured child needs to experience successful communication. Where the child is showing signs of distress or frustration it is particularly important to ensure that he has plenty of opportunities to succeed. While the child remains unable to use speech reliably for communication the priority should remain the promotion of functional communication, rather than the rehabilitation of specific linguistic skills.

Acquired childhood aphasia

Speech and language difficulties caused by traumatic brain injury in child-hood are known as 'acquired childhood aphasias.' The most common features of this disorder, which is associated with loss or disturbance of speech, language, and communication skills occurring after a period of normal language development, are described by Murdoch (1990) as: 'initial *mutism* followed by a period of *reduced speech initiative*; a *non-fluent speech output; simplified syntax; impaired auditory comprehension* abilities; an *impairment in naming; dysarthria;* and *disturbances in reading and writing'*.

It is only once the child begins to show some signs of recovery that the nature of any specific speech and language difficulties may become apparent.

Mutism

Following brain injury, many children have a period of mutism where they appear unable to use spoken language and are often unable or reluctant to communicate using alternative methods. Some children remain silent, although appearing to have some understanding and they may be progressing well in other aspects of recovery. The reason for this period of mutism is not well understood but it may persist for some time; the lack of spontaneous speech is often the greatest cause of concern to the child's parents and carers.

Reduced speech initiative

Alternatively, the child may be able to speak but lack the motivation to do so. Such children will often give short or monosyllabic answers to direct questions and may be able to repeat words and phrases on request, but do not spontaneously initiate speech.

Non-fluency

Children with acquired childhood aphasias, particularly in the earlier phases of recovery, typically produce spoken language which is slow, effortful, and lacking the normal prosodic features of speech.

Simplified syntax

As the child begins to use more spoken language, disturbances of syntax may become apparent. Often the child will simplify the grammatical structure of his sentence, so that it resembles that of a much younger child. For example, 'When Mum come?' rather than 'When *is my* Mum com*ing*?', with the child tending to use the content items, i.e. words which have a concrete meaning, and omit the function words and word-endings, i.e. those which primarily affect the grammatical structure of the sentence. Overt grammatical errors do occur but tend to be less common than simplifications.

Impaired auditory comprehension

While the child's difficulties with spoken language are clearly apparent, problems with the understanding of spoken language are less obvious. However, it is important that the child's auditory comprehension, i.e. his ability to understand spoken language, is assessed in an objective manner rather than assumed from his general state of responsiveness. Parents are often adamant that their child has good understanding, but unfortunately receptive language skills are frequently impaired in the severely brain-injured child.

Impaired naming

Word-finding or naming deficits are a common feature of acquired childhood aphasia and result in the child being unable to select the specific word he requires. These problems result in the child selecting the wrong word, which may be an item from the same semantic group, e.g. 'cat' for 'dog' or one which sounds similar, e.g. 'doll' for 'dog'. Alternatively, the child may use a non-specific word, e.g. 'animal', 'thingy', or give a description, e.g. 'It goes woof woof '. Naming difficulties can be frustrating for both the child, who may have some awareness of his errors, and his carers as it reduces the child's ability to communicate successfully and can therefore also affect his confidence.

Dysarthria

"Dysarthria is a collective name for a group of related speech disorders that are due to disturbances in muscular control of the speech mechanism resulting from impairment of any of the basic motor processes involved in the execution of speech" (Darley *et al* 1975).

The specific type of dysarthria encountered in the individual brain-injured child varies, but breath control for speech, voice quality, articulation, and the prosody or 'tune' of the voice may all be affected.

Reading and writing difficulties

Similar to the aphasias encountered in adults, acquired childhood aphasia is a disorder of processing and using language which can affect all modalities of language, i.e. speaking, understanding, reading, and writing. Disturbances of both reading and writing skills are common in acquired childhood aphasia and may persist in the child who appears to have made a good recovery. These problems therefore require careful management, in conjunction with teachers and educational psychologists, to minimize the impact on the child's educational progress.

MEDIUM TERM MANAGEMENT

Once the child is alert during the day and is managing to communicate his basic needs, he is becoming ready for more formal work aimed at improving specific speech and language skills. Children with brain injury can present with a complex range of difficulties and may pass through a phase of fairly rapid recovery during which constant reassessment and evaluation of therapeutic goals is essential.

All professionals involved with the child, as well as his parents, need to be aware of every aspect of the child's language impairment so that the focus of their concern is not purely his difficulties with, or lack of, spoken language. While difficulties with spoken language are the most obvious to the child and his parents, receptive difficulties often underlie the child's expressive problems, and therefore the importance of addressing any problems the child has with understanding cannot be overstated.

In the early stages of recovery, the child with impaired comprehension is likely to make use of situational cues to support his poor understanding of spoken language. Such cues are important props for the child and while he should not be discouraged from using them, it is important to ensure that his difficulties in understanding speech in the absence of such cues do not go unrecognized. For example, the child may open his mouth in response to someone holding out his toothbrush and saying 'Open your mouth', but cues in the situation, such as the presence of the toothbrush and the knowledge that toothbrushing always follows mealtimes, help the child to respond appropriately and enable him to give the impression of understanding without necessarily following any of the spoken language used. Older children and those with relatively intact cognitive skills can quickly learn compensatory strategies, thereby becoming adept at hiding their difficulties with spoken language.

Where the child shows evidence of auditory comprehension deficits, he will require specific therapeutic intervention designed to extend his understanding of spoken language. Comprehension difficulties need to be tackled in a systematic manner so that the child can see that he is making progress and his motivation to improve further is maintained.

All of the therapists' interactions with the child provide the opportunity to demonstrate to parents and other carers how the child can be encouraged to use his existing communication skills and strategies in simple everyday activities. It is particularly important for parents to see that it is possible to have good and useful communicative interactions with children who are unable to speak. In addition, as the speech and language therapist's intervention needs to address both the child's receptive and expressive language difficulties, the importance of modifying the complexity of language used when speaking *to* the child needs to be stressed. Parents need to be reassured that with help their child's understanding will improve and the use of strategies to promote comprehension, such as simplification of sentence structures, repetition, and allowing enough time for him to process information, need to be clearly and consistently demonstrated.

Activities which support the child's ability to use non-verbal communication skills can be helpful in restoring his confidence in his ability to communicate. For the very young child, 'therapy' needs to be placed in the context of play so that the child is encouraged to engage in everyday play activities. Pretend play activities such as putting a doll to bed, feeding toy animals, etc. can be used even with children who have limited physical skills. For example, the child can be encouraged to choose to put either a doll or teddy to bed by pointing at the appropriate toy, and then go through a bedtime routine, selecting the required items through pointing. Where the child is physically unable to perform the actions, he can instruct the therapist with points or gestures or be encouraged to respond to 'yes' / 'no' questions. The therapist can demonstrate the use of open questions, i.e. those which do not have a fixed reply (e.g. 'I wonder what teddy wants to do next?'), to give the child the opportunity to influence the situation and develop his functional communication skills.

Older children require the same calm and relaxed approach, incorporating more age appropriate activities, although clearly these need to fall within the child's current range of ability. The use of natural gestures and facial expression, as well as any AAC system, should continue to be encouraged and all those involved in the child's care need to allow the child enough time to use such methods of communication, despite the fact that this is undoubtedly time-consuming.

Simple card games such as 'lotto' and 'pairs' are useful in that the child can play the game without needing to speak, but they provide a good opportunity for use of single words in an appropriate context (i.e. picture naming), which can be useful as the child begins to use some spoken language. Where the child is physically unable to manipulate cards, he can be encouraged to practise other skills such as eye-pointing as a natural component of the same activity. A wide variety of picture-based materials suitable for all age groups are now commercially available.

As well as using open questions, the therapist can also demonstrate the use of questions which provide the child with the opportunity to use his 'yes' or 'no' signals or, where the child is beginning to speak, 'forced alternatives' which give the child options, e.g. 'Shall we put it away ... or play again?', and therefore help the child to make simple verbal responses without his having to select the vocabulary and construct the phrase unaided. As with all activities, with the brain-injured child it is important to pause to allow him time to respond as the child may require additional time to process the information and formulate a response.

One of the most frustrating periods for parents during the process of their child's recovery can occur once the child has begun to make some communicative vocalizations, say an occasional word or been heard to use some spoken language. The child may not, however, use speech consistently to indicate his needs or ask for help despite *apparently* having some potential to do so. Parents need to be discouraged from attempting to 'force' the child to speak. Comments such as 'You can't have it until you ask' do little but put the child under inappropriate and unnecessary pressure to perform. Parents can be helped by reminding them that if the child *could* speak, he *would* do so, i.e. the problem is not that the child is stubbornly refusing to speak, but that due to the brain damage he has suffered he is unable to do so. As with any task that is difficult, the child is far more likely to speak when he is calm and relaxed than when he is directly instructed to do so.

Again, one of the functions of the speech and language therapist is to reassure the parents that the child is not being lazy, but that this reduced-speech initiative is a symptom of the childs injury and that he can be helped by reducing rather than increasing the demands for spoken language placed upon him. It is also important that any AAC system the child has been using is not withdrawn as soon as he has uttered a single word. The selection of vocabulary and formation of sentences may still be difficult and so the alternative system should be left available to the child until he spontaneously ceases to use it. The child who becomes so 'dependent' on an AAC system that he continues to use it when it is genuinely no longer required has yet to be encountered, and in our experience, problems arise far more frequently from the withdrawal of systems for communication support at too early a stage in recovery.

It is important that as the child begins to use speech, adults continue to respond to the content of the speech rather than the fact that the child has spoken, and try to maintain a calm manner. Drawing attention to the child's speech output in the early days is likely to reduce, rather than increase, his speech output. It is also important for parents to realize that in the early stages of recovery the child's ability to say things can come and go. Therefore, just because the child may have said something once does not mean that a verbal reply to copious questions should immediately be insisted upon.

The importance of encouraging the child to communicate and responding to *what* he has 'said' rather than *how* he has said it cannot be overemphasized. Throughout the child's therapy, the therapist should stress the need to help the child regain the ability to communicate through providing him with real opportunities to do so. As the child begins to use more spoken language, difficulties with sentence construction may become apparent. By this stage the child should be able to cope with more structured therapeutic tasks and therefore programmes to address the child's specific difficulties can be devised.

Children who have experienced brain injuries often have difficulty generalizing skills; the child may demonstrate his ability to perform a specific task in a structured situation, e.g. greet someone appropriately, but may not actually do this in a 'real' situation. It is therefore important that generalization tasks, which help the child to practise and use the skills he has learnt in 'real' situations, are built into the programme and that there is close liaison between the child's teachers as well as his parents, to ensure that the child has the necessary support and encouragement in the use of new skills.

Maintaining the child's motivation is not always easy but trying to ensure that tasks are based on materials that he finds interesting, as well as providing concrete methods of demonstrating success, can often be helpful.

In young children, simple naming activities will often reveal evidence of word finding difficulties with phrases such as 'a thingy' and 'Mum's got one' being common. Simple sorting and categorizing activities, as well as tasks involving immediate recall such as remembering all the things in dolly's bag, are activities which can easily be practised throughout the day. Once the child's parents have understood the principles behind this type of task they can adapt it as appropriate to different experiences throughout the child's day. Older children also benefit from categorizing and immediate-recall activities. In addition, they can also be encouraged to participate in word generating games such as recalling animal names, TV programmes, or thinking of words beginning with a given letter. Using a stop watch and giving time limits can be motivating for some children and can also be helpful in giving the child clear evidence that he is making progress.

Cueing strategies, i.e. those strategies which help a child to retrieve a given word, vary from individual to individual. Gestures are often helpful, particularly early on where the range of words attempted is more limited. Forced alternatives are usually the easiest, with semantic cues (e.g. 'something you drink from') and phonemic cues (e.g. 'it starts with "c" ') more difficult.

Older children can be helped to self-cue; for example, where the child has some literacy skills, the use of these to assist with word-finding can be explored, e.g. by looking at an alphabet card or going through the alphabet in their head some children will be able to generate their own phonemic cues. Some children can cue themselves by visualizing either the item or the written word. Strategies which help one child will not necessarily help another and the most effective cueing strategies for each individual will need to be established.

Assessment

Informal assessment provides the therapist with an impression of the child's functional communication skills. The therapist can gain a great deal of information from observing how the child communicates with those around him and noting any areas of difficulty or sources of frustration. For example, when visitors arrive, does the child greet them appropriately and respond to simple questions? How does he communicate his basic needs such as pain and discomfort, hunger, simple requests, etc.? If the child uses any spoken language, is this intelligible, and if he does not speak, does he use appropriate non-verbal communication?

The non-verbal responses of the child are also important. For example, does he make eye contact with the speaker, smile, and use facial expressions appropriately, etc.? For children using any type of alternative/augmentative system it is important to establish how efficiently the child can use the system for purposeful communication.

Assessing the child's ability to respond appropriately to simple conversational speech provides the therapist with useful information about the child's functional abilities and helps with the planning of further assessment and intervention. A more structured assessment of the child's level of understanding is, however, also required. For example, can he point to body parts, familiar objects or pictures on request, follow simple instructions or a sequence of requests? Assessment of the child's ability to respond to the spoken language only is essential, but where the child is clearly unable to demonstrate consistent understanding, establishing how much he can be helped by gestures and other non-verbal cues is crucial in helping those working with the child to communicate successfully with him.

Once the child becomes stable, standardized assessment is important for identifying his level of ability in order to inform current management, monitor progress, and highlight areas of specific difficulty. A comprehensive assessment of receptive and expressive language skills is essential, but there are very few assessment tools designed specifically for the brain injured child. This lack of specific assessment tools for children with acquired childhood aphasias means that the therapist often has to rely on tests designed either for children with developmental difficulties, which may not highlight the specific problems of the brain-injured child, or for adults with acquired speech and language disorders, where the materials may not be particularly attractive or appropriate for young children. In addition, assessment materials designed for use with adults may also utilize written language skills which the young child will not yet have developed.

The Children's Aphasia Screening Test (Whurr and Evans 1986) provides some basic information about the child's ability to perform some simple tasks such as object and picture matching and identification, confrontation naming and serial speech and may be useful in providing a baseline measure of ability. However, the child who is making a reasonable recovery will soon reach the ceiling level on this test. Tests which provide more detailed information about the childs abilities and areas of difficulty are therefore required.

A description of the full range of assessments available and which may be suitable for any individual child with ACA is beyond the scope of this chapter, and therefore only a small number, which have been found to be particularly useful with this population are described in the text. However, further information is widely available from other sources. e.g. Kersner (1992).

Comprehension

Difficulties in the understanding of spoken language are a common feature in children with brain injuries. The severity of the problem is variable but few children escape without at least some degree of higher level comprehension deficit.

Assessment of comprehension skills usually involves the child listening to a word or sentence and selecting the picture to represent this from a small number of pictures on the page. Thus the child's understanding is assessed without his having to make any verbal response. For the child who has significant physical involvement, it is important to establish responses he can make easily and reliably. Liaison with the child's physiotherapist may be helpful in establishing a reliable motor response or the child may be taught to use eye-pointing or scanning techniques. The necessary reliance on visual stimuli in assessment makes evaluation of the child with significant visual problems particularly difficult.

Full assessment should include evaluation of the child's ability to understand both sentence structure and vocabulary. For the young child, developmental assessments of comprehension are helpful in establishing his level of understanding, i.e. comparing his understanding of spoken language to that of his peers. TROG – the Test for the Reception of Grammar (Bishop 1989) provides a tool for assessing the child's understanding of specific grammatical structures.

A number of assessments of children's understanding of vocabulary are now available. The British Picture Vocabulary Scale (Dunn *et al* 1982) is widely used, although this can take some time to complete. The receptive-language subtests of the Test of Word Knowledge (TOWK) (Wiig and Secord 1992) are particularly useful especially when compared with the expressive scales of the same test, described below, to indicate any discrepancy between receptive and expressive ability, as measured on the same scale. The receptive language subtests of the Clinical Evaluation of Language Fundamentals – Revised Edition (Semel *et al*. 1988) are also useful for highlighting specific areas of deficit, particularly in the child with higher level problems, and especially now that UK rather than American norms are available. (CELF-R^{UK}) UK adaptation – National Hospitals College of Speech Science (1994).

Expressive language difficulties

Lack of spoken language can be an extremely frustrating problem for both the child and his carers, particularly where he is making good progress in other areas and there is no obvious, specific cause for the lack of speech.

As the child begins to use some speech or to use an AAC system at a level complex enough to require the use of novel combinations of words and phrases, the therapist will begin to be able to make some assessments of any expressive difficulties.

For a thorough, formal assessment of a child's expressive language skills the expressive language subtests of the CELF-R^{UK} are ideal. The subtests cover a variety of expressive language skills, providing a detailed picture of the child's abilities and areas of particular difficulty. However, this takes some time to administer and requires a reasonable degree of cooperation and concentration from the child, and may therefore be considered most appropriate for highlighting areas of residual deficit in the child who is making a good recovery, as well as a tool for measuring changes over time.

As quick, easily administered screening tools, the Action Picture Test (Renfrew 1989) and the Bus Story (Renfrew 1991), which involve answering a series of structured questions about a set of pictures and retelling a simple story respectively, provide a basic measure of the child's ability to form sentences and to convey information, and can then be repeated as a basic measure of progress. For older children for whom these materials are inappropriate, similar non-standardized tasks can be devised, based on the same principles.

Word finding

Word-finding difficulties are extremely common in brain-injured children. Thus, even during the relatively early stages of rehabilitation, time spent on word-retrieval activities and teaching cueing strategies to both the child and his carers is useful.

Confrontation naming (i.e. asking the child to name a series of objects or pictures presented to him) is commonly used to assess the child's expressive vocabulary and/or any word-finding difficulties. Particularly in older children, word-finding problems may be detected only on attempting to perform such a task, as the child may be able to successfully conceal his difficulties during spontaneous conversation. During non-standardized naming activities the speech and language therapist can assess the child's response to different types of help, for example, gestures or semantic and phonemic cues as described above.

The Word-finding Vocabulary Scale (Renfrew 1988), which is a picture-based test of confrontation naming, provides a quick screening assessment of word-finding abilities in the young child, but does not incorporate any qualitative information such as any strategies the child may use or find helpful. The expressive scales of the Test Of Word Knowledge (TOWK) (Wiig and Secord 1992) and the Test of Word Finding (German 1986) take longer to administer but provide more detailed qualitative and quantitative information.

Reading and writing problems

As all modalities of language may be affected in acquired childhood aphasia, although not necessarily to the same degree, many children will have some disturbance of reading and writing skills. The underlying nature of the child's difficulty, for example difficulty with the segmental skills required to break a word up into its constituent parts for spelling, poor memory, visuo-spatial problems, etc., need to be established so that appropriate intervention can be planned. A variety of professionals may have expertise in the management of specific aspects of the problems of reading and writing, including for example, teachers, educational psychologists, and occupational therapists, as well as speech and language therapists, and careful liaison and cooperation is therefore particularly essential.

LONG TERM MANAGEMENT

At one time, children with acquired childhood aphasia were thought to make virtually complete recoveries. However, it is now clear that this is not the case and many children have residual difficulties which significantly affect their educational progress; 'It is probable that few children can really be said to make a complete recovery from ACA' (Lees 1993). The persistence of language difficulties into adulthood has also been clearly described (Jordan and Murdoch 1994). In addition, the child may have other difficulties arising from his injury and continue to require the support of a variety of different professionals. Any difficulties the child has with speech and language skills must continue to be viewed in the context of his other abilities, particularly cognitive and motor skills as well as his individual social and emotional needs. Careful consideration still needs to be given to the coordination of the child's management, particularly if he returns to mainstream education.

Problems with the understanding and processing of information delivered at speed, particularly for the child who has the short term memory deficit often associated with brain injury, can have a huge influence on the child's ability to cope in mainstream education. Children and their teachers need to be taught to use strategies to help with the understanding and retention of information, for example, breaking it down into more manageable 'chunks', making lists of key points, etc. Specific strategies for tackling word-finding problems, including the use of word processors where appropriate, can help the child learn to manage his residual deficits.

In addition, many children have persistent difficulties with the pragmatic or functional aspects of language. For example, they may have difficulty understanding figurative language, relying on literal interpretation and failing to understand jokes or colloquial expressions.

Expressively, the head-injured child may have similar difficulties, reflecting a lack of awareness of the social aspects of communication. Thus the child may express his thoughts literally, lacking the ability to modify his language in consideration of the listener's feelings.

Such difficulties can have a subtle effect on the child's ability to interact with his peers, thus influencing the child's reintegration to his local school and community.

The problems of the child with acquired childhood aphasia remain complex and poorly understood by the professionals attempting to treat them. A great deal of further work in this field is required to enable speech and language therapists and other professionals to address the particular needs of the child with non-traumatic, but particularly traumatic brain injury, and to help him to realize his full potential.

REFERENCES

Barrett, J. and Herriotts, P. (1995). *Communication aids and access to computer technology*. The Disability Information Trust, Oxford.

Bishop, D.V.M. (1989). *TROG – the test for the reception of grammar*. University of Manchester. Distributed by the author.

Darley, F.L., Aronson, A.E., and Brown, J.R. (1975). *Motor speech disorders*. W.B. Saunders Co., Philadelphia.

Dunn, L. M., Whetton, C., and Pintilie, D. (1982). *The British picture vocabulary scale*. NFER-Nelson, Windsor.

German, D. J. (1986). *Test of word-finding* . Taskmaster Ltd; Leicester.

Jordan, F. M. and Murdoch, B. E. (1994). Severe closed head injury in childhood: linguistic outcomes into adulthood. *Brain Injury*, 8, 501–8.

Kersner, M. (1992) *Tests of voice, speech, and language*. Whurr Publishers Ltd; London.

Kiernan, C., and Reid, B. (1987) *The pre-verbal communication schedule*. NFER-Nelson; Windsor.

Lees, J. A. (1993). *Children with acquired aphasias*. Whurr Publishers Ltd; London.

Murdoch, (1990), B.E. Acquired aphasia in childhood. In *Acquired Speech and Language Disorders*. (ed. B. E. Murdoch). Chapman and Hall; London.

Renfrew, C. E. (1988). *Word-finding vocabulary scale*. Winslow Press, Bicester.

Renfrew, C. E. (1989) *The action picture test*. Winslow Press, Bicester.

Renfrew, C. E. (1991) *The bus story - a test of continuous speech*. Winslow Press, Bicester.

Whurr, R. and Evans, S. (1986). *The children's aphasia screening test*. Whurr Publishers Ltd, London.

Semel, E., Wiig, E. H., and Secord, W. (1987). *Clinical evaluation of language fundamentals - revised edition*. UK Adaptation (CELF-R[UK]) (UK adaptation – National Hospitals College of Speech Science 1994). Harcourt Brace Jovanovich, New York.

Wiig, E. H., and Secord, W. (1992). *Test Of Word Knowledge (TOWK)*. The Psychological Corporation. Harcourt Brace Jovanovich, New York.

Computer programs

Mayer-Johnson. *Boardmaker*. Distributed by Don Johnson Special Needs, Warrington.

8

Cognitive deficits

Tony Baldwin, Heather Seddon, Colin Demellweek,
Bronwen Hughes and Sue Fishwick

INTRODUCTION

The purpose of this chapter is to give a basic outline of the cognitive and
educational difficulties which may follow an acquired brain injury. The focus
of the chapter will be on traumatic brain injuries as these tend to be more
frequently associated with long-term educational problems, which may often
be subtle and become apparent only some months or years following the
injury. As with other chapters there is considerable overlap with additional
problems – including speech and language impairment and emotional and
behavioural difficulties – which again reinforces the need for a coordinated
and multidisciplinary approach for these children.

As the number of children surviving head injuries grows, there is an
increasing recognition of the complexity that acquired cognitive deficits
can take. Children who are unfortunate enough to suffer a brain injury
are frequently able to make a good physical recovery, and this can mask a
range of cognitive deficits that may severely interfere with functional living
and educational skills. Sometimes the cognitive deficits are quite apparent,
but frequently they are subtle and can easily be confused with behavioural or
personality factors. This is particularly evident when a child's ability to learn
new tasks is impaired. Whereas many children have significant and long term
initial disabilities, it is not uncommon to find children making pleasing
recovery in which old skills return, and after some intensive rehabilitation
they will almost be able to function at their pre-morbid level. Unfortunately
they may find the ability to learn, acquire, memorise and cope with the
general demands within normal learning situations extremely difficult. New
learning becomes ever more difficult for them and their difficulties can be
underestimated by those working with them. The necessity for more systematic and long term follow up of brain-injured children, was raised by
Oddy (1993).

These difficulties with new learning may not be so apparent for those
working within the adult field, because after leaving school the last complex
skill to be acquired usually by most adults is learning to drive. We all

experience the difficulties of working out how a new microwave or video recorder works, and frequently it is the children in the family who can use such equipment before the adults. This gives us one indication of how learning new skills can become increasingly difficult with age, and yet the problem is relatively unseen since we all hold a body of knowledge and skills that make us able to function quite adequately in daily living and society. However, young children are only in the very formative years of the educational process and many years of learning lie ahead. Children are in a competing and comparative situation in which their rate of progress is, to some extent, dictated by others. Since they are usually working within a group of children of a similar age their ability to cope at a crude level is made by comparison with their ability to cope with their peers. For a child who can not keep up with his peers, there is a gradual slowing and falling behind, and this affects not only his educational standing but also his own self-esteem. Fortunately there has been considerable enlightenment during recent years towards providing children with a curriculum that has been differentiated/ modified to meet their own particular needs. This has in large been brought on by the greater recognition and integration of children who have special educational needs into mainstream education and the requirements of the 1981 and 1993 Education Acts. Whereas there are many sound and good examples of this working in practice it is often difficult to achieve on account of the time required and the numbers of children who require such programmes. The need for a greater understanding of head injuries in the educational system has been well expressed by Johnson (1992), who outlined the need for a greater awareness of the nature of the learning difficulties such children can face.

A further aspect of brain injury in children is the so called 'sleeper effect'. Sometimes, a child can make what appears to be good recovery with no obvious difficulties in the first few years following the injury. However, as the child approaches adolescence, particularly in the transfer from a junior school to a secondary school, the hidden difficulties may become apparent when a higher order of learning skills are required. It is, therefore, not uncommon to find children returning to their old mainstream schools and coping for one, two, or even three years, before then failing and falling behind their peers.

NATURE OF INJURY

In the majority of cases, the extent of a learning difficulty resulting from a head or other brain injury is related to the severity and nature of the head injury (Levin *et al*. 1982). For instance, in a child whose brain injury had been complicated by severe cerebral oedema (brain swelling), the supply of blood and oxygen to the brain may be severely compromised. This causes diffuse damage, and on recovery, general cognitive functioning can be impaired. Frequently, it is not an obvious impairment but more of a general slowing of mental processing. The child's short-term memory is not quite as good as it once was, and his ability to think, react, and formulate ideas is slower and not as acute as it had been previously. Sometimes this has been referred to as 'living in the slow lane' (Johnson *et al.* 1989). The child with pre-existing problems appears to cope even less well in these circumstances, and, understandably, any pre-existing disability may be exaggerated. Therefore it is not unusual to find that a child who had some memory problems before the injury has them in much more exaggerated form following the injury. The same is also true for the child with attentional and concentration difficulties.

REHABILITATION

The age at which a head injury occurs is an important factor to be taken into account when considering the potential implications of any acquired brain damage. Very young children appear to have a remarkable ability to compensate and cope with a wide range of difficulties, and this is particularly the case if the child was bright and able before the head injury. Obviously, if the child has been very severely injured then he may always require a great deal of intensive support. More subtle injuries may render children less able than they were, but they frequently remain sufficiently able to cope within the context of a normal learning environment, although often very specific learning difficulties may become apparent in the course of time.

The cognitive demands that are placed on children do vary considerably throughout their lives. Within the context of an infant or primary school the day is structured, there is a degree of routine, material is prepared for them, and they are directed to activities. There is a major change when children transfer to the secondary school as they are now in a learning environment where they have to take far greater responsibility for themselves. The day has to be planned, books or equipment have to be got ready, and they have to be able to switch from one activity to another, usually within the space of a forty-minute lesson. It is under these circumstances that the child with a brain injury frequently comes to grief, as the system demands a high degree of organization and planning and the ability to switch mental set and thinking processes. Being in the right place at the right time with the right equipment requires a considerable amount of effort and is a skill that can elude many children.

Generally speaking, within the educational system there is no differentiation between children who have acquired neurological deficits and those whose problems arise out of developmental disorders. There is no reported research from literature that would tell us how these groups are different, although a number of authors, including Cruickshank *et al* (1961), do consider their specific needs. Brain-injured children do often learn somewhat differently from other children. They can be more impulsive or hyperactive and distractible, and the discrepancies between their ability levels and performance can be more extreme. Whereas some learning deficits may be very specific, others may be hardly affected, and therefore the child with subtle and complex difficulties has problems coping with an educational system that can very often group children into some overall concept of ability. The onvious need for the greater recognition and provision of some form of specialist service/tution for brain injured children was well expressed by Telzrow (1987). This paper was written outlining core issues that should be addressed in the educational rehabilitation programmes. Unfortunately in recent years the educational system has become totally curriculum led following the introduction of the national curriculum. This has made the implication of any wider rehabilitation programs in the educational setting extremely difficult to effect. Even though there is the option for the national curriculum to be disapplied most schools are reluctant to make such provision.

The brain-injured child may have a reliance on learning strategies and styles that were developed before the head injury. Whereas these may have been entirely successful in the past, this may no longer be the case, and old habits can die hard. He may also retain the pre-injury self-concept of a normal child, who may have been one of the best in class, who found work relatively easy, and was used to success. In a few brief weeks he has been reduced to a child who struggles to retain information, and only with very considerable effort is he able to learn. He therefore sees a progressive sliding down the class hierarchy at a time when self-esteem may already be affected due to physical injuries or changes in behaviour, or both.

Rehabilitation of the child is usually directed towards a gradual recovery back into, what could be loosely termed, 'a normal lifestyle'. Areas of specific deficit are addressed. However, much depends on the relevance of the assessments that are carried out, and therefore, the aims of any rehabilitation programme. We view rehabilitation as creating an environment in which the child is allowed to recover, and in which areas of deficit are retrained by teaching strategies and compensatory mechanisms in order to help the child cope with any cognitive deficits. There is also the necessity to consider the creation or manipulation of the child's environment in order to allow him to function more adequately, and this obviously may mean a change of schooling.

When considering the forms of intervention we can divide them up in five stages.

Firstly, there is the period of spontaneous recovery that occurs. Therefore, the aim of the rehabilitation may be to facilitate the child in that recovery to maintain the motivation, interest, and perseverance and allow him to advance by providing him with the appropriate progression of tasks, in order that he can engage and cope with skills at increasingly higher levels.

Secondly, it may be necessary to retrain the child, giving him alternative cognitive styles or methods of processing information in order that he can cope with more complex tasks. This is usually carried out when it is realized that spontaneous recovery is slowing and there is a need to provide the child with strategies to cope with higher-level skills.

Thirdly, there is the need to develop the functional skills and to try and encourage normalization and generalization of skills within the everyday environment that the child is likely to encounter.

Fourthly, environmental changes have to be considered; it may be that the child cannot return to the normal learning environment and therefore the difficulties of readapting and accepting longer term disabilities may have to be faced.

Fifthly, if the child continues to have learning problems and possibly also physical difficulties, there is the issue of helping him come to terms with the changes in his life and to readjust to his new concept of himself.

Needless to say, throughout this process the child's parents need constant reassurance, support, and guidance.

ASSESSMENT

It is often only in a neuropsychological assessment that the underlying cognitive deficits of children who have sustained a brain injury become apparent. Whereas significant and global deficits are immediately apparent, subtle problems may not be obvious or looked for, especially if they follow a mild head injury (Bawden *et al* 1985). The recognition that subtle acquired deficits can affect academic performance and prove quite persistent has been noted by those working with such children (Wrightson *et al* 1995). The identification of many specific deficits may not be revealed in a general intellectual assessment and it has to be recalled that intelligence tests measure a collection of skills, including attention, motor performance and motor and processing speed. Indeed, as Lezak [1988] suggests, the concept of IQ in many respects is an outdated one and certainly it must be used with caution when making any assumptions about the brain-injured child. It is useful as an indicator of levels of functioning and can be used as a basis from which further testing can be carried out, but it is only an initial screening test in which a broader and more detailed neuropsychological assessment can take place. Arguably the best source of general information on neuropsychological assessments is to be found in Lezak (1995) but this relates to adults.

There are several neuropsychological test batteries that have been developed for use with children and which attempt to provide a comprehensive neuropsychological assessment. These have been downward extensions of adult tests. The Nebraska Neuropsychological Battery for Children was based on Luria's theoretical model of brain functioning (Golden 1981). The Halstead–Reitan test is probably the most widely used test in the United States. There are two child versions of this test available, for children in the age groups 9 to 14 and a version for children aged 5 to 8.

The Wechsler Intelligence Scale for children (1992), – has probably become the most widely used individual test of general intelligence and a considerable amount has been written relating to the profiles obtained (Kaufman 1994). Unfortunately it was often the case that too much emphasis was placed on the overall IQ result in the past. The test does have an inherent validity especially if all the 12 sub-tests are administered. Analysis of the results is then able to yield a verbal quotient (which gives an indication of the child's ability to reason with words, learn verbal material and process verbal information) and a performance quotient (which gives an indication of the child's ability to process non verbal information including non verbal reasoning). The additional information available from the provision of the four additional Index Quotients of Verbal Comprehension, Perceptual Organisation, Freedom from Distraction and Processing Speed, has proved valuable in providing a basis for helping to identify areas of comparative weakness and specific deficits. These patterns do need to be interpreted with caution as they lack a prescriptive and predictive value in the assessment of brain damage however they do provide a valuable indicator from which further assessments can be made. The test has sometimes been used inappropriately to confirm not only the presence of a brain impairment, but also the lateralization and localization of impairment. Too much reliance on comparison of verbal/performance scales can also miss more subtle and specific deficits with some children not uncommonly showing significant processing and learning problems despite having a normal IQ score.

Whereas a full cognitive assessment may be a starting point in the assessment of the brain injured child a great deal of information can be obtained using an hypothesis testing and problem-solving approach looking at functional skills and deficits. This can then be supplemented using a range of neuropsychological assessment tools that are available and these are well described by Strauss and Spreen (1991). Unfortunately, many of the tests have been devised for adults and although child norms are available they tend to be derived from very small numbers, and the tests themselves may not hold an inherent interest for children. A further complication of the neuropsychological assessment of children is that subtle deficits can be acquired in the child's formative years which may initially appear insignificant and yet affect the child's long term potential. Reitan (1981) found that children sustaining damage at the age of four years showed a distinctly different learning curve from older children with brain damage. Complex skills may not be expected of children in their formative years, and therefore deficits acquired early on in a child' life may not become significant until much later in their lives. Consequently, there is the need for the opportunity to carry out regular reviews of the child's progress.

The basis of any treatment programme must therefore take into account the neuropsychological deficits in children as these will influence the child's learning style and identify the nature of their specific learning difficulties. Assessments are therefore broadly based and not restricted to a basic IQ figure. At the same time there has to be recognition that individual tests that are considered to be sensitive to brain impairment are often evaluating a range of skills, hence their sensitivity, but they are not necessarily assessing a specific area of functioning. Whereas some information may be derived from specific tests, valuable information can be derived from detailed observation of the child in normal situations. This type of functional assessment augmenting a formal assessment model was advocated by Milton *et al.* (1991). A comprehensive neuropsychological evaluation should therefore sample the following range of attributes which may or may not have been provided by other professionals:

1. The child's physical skills need to be considered. At a fine motor level this includes an assessment of the child's functional living skills including dressing, feeding and their educational implications. Evaluation of the child's gross motor skills include the child's functional mobility within the home and school, and his ability to take part in recreation sports.

2. An evaluation of the child's sensory and perceptual skills and the implications. Dysfunction of vision, hearing or touch may have occurred and this can result in an impairment of localisation and/or recognition of stimuli. Any impairment, be it a partial loss, or simply a distortion can significantly affect the child's ability to learn.

3. An assessment of the child's overall intellectual functioning using some standardized assessment. This would usually include an assessment that would provide some profile of the child's skills looking at areas of comparative strengths and weaknesses and thereby providing an informed basis on which to plan further detailed testing and from which the significance of other assessments can be evaluated.

4. Assessment of the child's basic educational skills is essential and this includes not only reading accuracy and spelling skills but also (and this is of fundamental importance), the child's reading comprehension as frequently it is comprehension skills that are impaired following a brain injury. Mathematical skills are also commonly impaired, because of difficulties in mental processing or spatial awareness, or both.

5. An examination of the child's ability to attend to a given task, to think flexibly, and organize themselves – ie, his ability to cope with changing situations and problems. This includes an evaluation of the child's ability to solve problems in real life situations and make reasonable judgements given the information that would be available to him. Many of these skills are covered by the term executive functioning.

6. Memory is often an area that can be impaired following a brain injury and some assessment of the child's functional memory is needed either from questionnaires or functionally based tests. Deficits in short term memory in particular can lead to difficulties with verbal comprehension.

7. Some assessment of the child's ability to process information efficiently and quickly is required. The brain-injured child may have difficulties in the rate at which he can process many tasks and this can cause difficulties in a range of situations from the ability to follow normal playground activities to the ability to keep up with both the verbal and written tasks presented in class.

8. Communication is a crucial skill which can frequently be impaired following a brain injury. Within the expressive domain it is necessary to look at the child's functional communications skills including intelligibility of speech, pragmatics and word-finding. Within the area of receptive language, the child's ability to understand short instructions and longer more complex conversation is needed. (This is discussed in more detail in Chapter 7).

9. Behavioural effects and changes in personality are a major factor relating to the child's social and educational rehabilitation. Emotional lability is

common and it is necessary to look at the child's ability to cope with the ups and downs of everyday life, including the frustration often encountered in the learning situation. The ability to inhibit the first impulse is necessary for both good social adaptation and learning.

It has to be appreciated that children do not follow a textbook pattern of acquired learning difficulty. Many children may appear to have returned to their pre-traumatic levels of functioning, but often more detailed assessment reveals a range of difficulties that may become more apparent or pronounced as time goes on. Often these residual impairments affect the child's functional skills both at an academic and social level. It is therefore necessary to look at a range of processing difficulties in the brain injured child. There is no one overall test or method of assessment that can evaluate all these aspects of functioning. Indeed in some cases, tests are not appropriate and we find that observational checklists can provide an excellent basis for some initial information, providing the observer knows what they are looking for. Given the rapid progress some children can make, the timing of any formal assessment can be variable and in the early stages assessments may best be done in the form of structured observations although detailed assessments will be required at some stage.

SENSORY AND PERCEPTUAL DEFICITS

Disorders of the sensory and perceptual system are possibly some of the most interesting and at times most difficult to fully quantify and identify. Whereas the complete loss of one area of sensory functioning will be obvious, subtle deficits can be acquired following a brain injury and thse can be problematic when attempting to identify and consider what their implications may have on daily living skills or the acquisition of educational attainments. Throughout the literature in neuropsychology, there are numerous examples of the unusual single case studies of individuals who hae had their perceptual system disturbed (Luria 1976). It is noted that this area of deficit can tend to be the 'hidden' difficulty.

Perceptual problems need to be identified as soon as possible following a brain injury as they can be misinterpreted as behavioural and can be hard to distinguish from some motor problems.

Functional assessments are therefore required during the early stages of recovery. A formal assessment comes later if appropriate, to establish objective results. Tests which can be used with this population include the Test of Visual Perceptual Skills (non-motor) (TVPS) (Gardner 1982) which determines a child's visual perceptual strengths and weaknesses. Additionally, the Developmental Test of Visual Motor Integration

(Beery 1989) which is a developmental sequence of 24 geometric forms to be copied with paper and pencil, can be used to help identify deficits. For the older child and young adult the relatively new Visual Object and Space Perception Battery is a valuable assessment tool. (Warrington and James 1991)

Before any assessment can be carried out, it is essential to take account of any sensory deficits the child may have eg, whether glasses/hearing aids are normally worn, the influeces of any motor impairment and the child's receptive and expressive langauge abilities. Should the child have difficulties in any of these areas then this will have to be taken into consideration during any assessments and treatment. If the child has motor impairments, it is necessary to ensure that any environmental adaptations have been made and good positioning is extremely important. If seated, it is essential to ensure that the child is well-supported. Finally it is important to endeavour to make the environment as distraction-free as possible.

When considering sensory and perceptual deficits we must look at the areas in which the deficits can take place, since by definition we are looking at sensory deficits ie senses of taste, smell, touch (somato/sensory), auditory and visual system may be implicated either in isolation or in combination. A full review of these is to be found in Ellis and Young (1988).

Visual

Disorders in the visual system have received extensive coverage in the literature. When considering the visual system, we have to recognize that it is far more complex than the other senses. Whereas a partial loss of sensory function can appear simple, within the visual system, following a head injury there can be very specific losses in the visual fields and these can cause a range of functional difficulties for the child. For instance a loss of the lower visual field can result in a child who has great difficulty coming downstairs or coping with the uneven ground in the playground. Similarly the loss of a right or left sided visual field can result in an abnormal stance. The child apparently looking to the left or right of the speaker or the work that is being completed in an attempt to compensate for the loss of vision on one side or the other. Such an abnormal stance can result in social difficulties as other children do become somewhat perturbed if the normal reciprocal eye contact is not made. In the earliest stages of recovery, it is necessary to first assess the child's visual attention, and ability to focus and maintain gaze on an object moving slowly from the periphery to mid line. It is important to ascertain what gains the child's visual attention (nb when testing for this, the tester must be aware of excluding other factors, ie not wearing visually distracting clothing with stripes, not using toys that make sounds and not using his voice.)

Disorders of the visual perceptual system have long been held as one of the factors causing children to have learning difficulties and the Frostig Test (1966) was used extensively in the late 60s to early 70s. It does follow that a child who had difficulties readily discriminating individual letters and word patterns on a page could have difficulties learning to read (although these are by no means the only cause). With children who have acquired brain injuries, deficits in visual perceptual skills are common and much of the prepared work and materials that are available are well-suited to this group.

The brain-injured child may have an inability to recognize objects within a visual field (although the deficits may also arise from word finding difficulties). Some interesting work does show the specificity of this deficit eg facial recognition, where the individuals cannot recognize familiar faces, which is known as prosopagnosia. Such difficulties can be established by asking parents whether the child recognizes them and other visitors facially. This can be extended to include recognition of familiar people in photographs. The child may be unable to name or use colours correctly, or they may have difficulties making sense of ambiguous material. If such problems exist the child can be given compensatory strategies using verbal prompts and encouraged to talk their way through the problem and look for helpful details.

Difficulties with spatial awareness and spatial judgement do appear to cause a number of quite significant difficulties, not only in day-to-day living but also within the educational context. At a functional level the child may have difficulties positioning himself in relationship to other objects (eg the child who cannot position him or herself in front/behind/next to another, when requested) or understanding and developing a good concept of his way around his environment.

There is an interesting deficit which we see following some head injuries, referred to as visual neglect, the ignoring of information usually to the left of them. It is seen in the early stages of recovery in some children and it tends not to be such a persistent problem as noted in adults. In cases where it does persist the child may need considerable prompting and training to scan to the left.

Visual motor disturbances have long been recognized as a problem leading to educational difficulties. The main area of difficulty, of course in this situation, is the child's ability to copy material accurately as in copying geometrical shapes, letters, diagrams etc. Such deficits are dealt with in detail in Chapter 5. In so far as they interfere with educational skills such as handwriting, we use a very structural teaching approach using verbal mediation as discussed later.

The child's ability to recognize the position of objects in space (ie their visual spatial relationship) and of objects in relation to themselves, can be disturbed following a brain injury. These skills are essential in everyday life (eg to ensure safety when crossing the roads and judging distance, direction, and depth).

'Figure ground perception' is a term used for the child's ability to distinguish foreground from background information. Such deficits can have quite a disabling effect, particularly when it comes to children working from some of the more highly illustrated work books, where type face can be written across quite complex artistic background work.

Auditory

Disorders in the auditory system are well recognized, ranging from the difficulties of phonological awareness and its relationship to reading skills (Goswomi and Bryant 1991), to the very unusual and fortunately quite rare disorder known as Landau-Kleffner Syndrome, where the child is able to hear sounds but cannot identify and interpret speech patterns. The neuropsychological model of speech perception has been an area that has received considerable attention in recent years. Problems in the area of auditory perception appear to have the main effect on compromising the child's literacy skills, although auditory perception in its own right can prove problematic at a functional level within a large classroom setting. Anyone who has recorded in such an environment realises the high level of ambient background noise that can hinder the accurate perception of what is being said. The child may be able to understand using contextual and situational cues and their knowledge of the subject to help them understand what is being said. This does place an additional load on the attentional system and in a child who may already have difficulties, it can significantly impair them at a functional level.

Tactile/somato - sensory

Problems in the area of tactile sensation, which includes the ability to identify objects by touch, appreciate temperature and pain and also the position of limbs in space (see also Chapter 5) – can be quite handicapping. Whereas deficits in this area of functioning can prove disabling to an adult, at least they can have the potential dangers explained to them. In young children further injuries and accidents may occur because of the lack of appreciation of pain, heat or where their hands are. Of course the relevance of being able to correctly identify objects by touch is well known, to those who search for objects without the use of vision when looking for coins in a pocket or trying to find a lightswitch or keyhole in the dark.

Olfactory/taste

There would appear to be very limited information available on how taste may be affected following a head injury and of course this is an area that is extremely difficult to quantify in children who may be unable to give an accurate description of what they are tasting. However, deficits in smell (olfaction) are well-recognized and are also more readily reported in adult literature although of course this problem is also seen in children. Such deficits at a functional level may not appear to cause the individual child any particular difficulty, although one can imagine situations where the loss of smell could be quite critical eg smoke, burning, decaying food, petrol etc.

INFORMATION PROCESSING

A common deficit arising from a brain injury, is the ability to process information at the normal rate. Whereas the child may be able to carry out a variety of mental tasks, the speed at which these are completed in a brain injured child may be significantly slower than it would be for a normal child (Brooks 1984). The deficit may involve the speed at which the child can understand the task involved, learn the material, retrieve it from memory, and carry out the mental processes involved. Deficits in this area can severely limit the ability of the child to function in many everyday situations, and deficits can arise following even a mild head injury (Wrightson *et al*, 1995). The child may find difficulty comprehending information at the normal rate, formulating his thoughts, and then carry-ing out the required actions. He may find it difficult to understand if too much information is presented on any one occasion. He may therefore initially start off understanding what is going on but rapidly lose his way as the amount of information accumulates. This is particularly the case if the level of information becomes more complex and can occur in the formal learning and social situation. In the teaching situation, this often shows itself in the child's inability to complete written assignments, or answer questions in the allotted time and therefore never being able to answer a question directed at the class as by the time he raises his hand someone else has answered before him.

Children who are significantly affected can find themselves severely disadvantaged at a social level. Whereas adults will give a child a sympa-thetic look and the necessary time to collect his thoughts, a more competitive adolescent group will not be so kind. In the playground the conversation moves on at the pace of the group so for those too slow to respond frequently find themselves left far behind – sometimes it is just easier not to try and the child may find himself becoming increasingly isolated from his peers. Johnson *et al.* (1989) refers to it as living in the slow lane.

The ability to understand and learn and then retrieve information involves a range of abilities, including attention, short-term memory, and the ability to manipulate the information in order to place it into a more permanent memory system. Essential to this is the ability to organize material into a meaningful manner so that it can be recalled and subsequently placed within some existing scheme or order. As Tromp and Mulder (1991) demonstrated, it is the access to the memory system which affects the speed at which information is processed. Information therefore has to be organized and categorized in order that it can be stored in some permanent memory system. In order to do this it is also necessary for the child to be able to distinguish between the core information or main ideas and differentiate this from any irrelevant information. It is apparent that a range of strategies can be used in this process. The rate, amount, and complexity of the material may exceed what the child can comfortably cope with. To help the child cope with such processing problems, an appreciation and understanding that they do have difficulties in this area of functioning is important in elevating some of the secondary emotional consequences of always being one step behind. It is then apparent that a range of strategies can be used in helping the child function more competently and improve their performance. Possibly the greatest assistance can be given by a simple review of the tasks that they are expected to complete. Whereas it is not possible to control the variables in playground activities, the organization of the tasks set either in class or at home can be considered and structured in such a manner as to lead them in a meaningful way through the problem.

If people are aware that the child may have these difficulties the problem can be partly resolved by altering the rate at which work is presented. It is also very valuable if the child can be given some strategies at a basic level to be able to say, 'Can you please explain that again?' 'Can you go through that a little slower, please?', or 'Can you let me think about that for a minute before I answer?'. These sort of responses can give the child a second opportunity to answer or resolve the problem and help to prevent an anxiety-producing situation from developing.

EXECUTIVE FUNCTIONING

One of the most vulnerable structures to be damaged in a head injury is that of the frontal lobes, and yet within the child literature it is only comparatively recently that interest is starting to be re-expressed in this crucial area of functioning. It was often assumed that frontal-lobe functioning was not particularly relevant to children's development, but this view is now changing. A recent review of development assessment of 'executive functioning' was made by Kelly *et al* (1996).

There is increasing evidence to suggest that frontal lobe development is crucial to many aspects of behaviour in early childhood. The terms 'frontal lobe functioning' and 'executive functioning' are now quite often used interchangeably although strictly speaking executive functioning does involves other attributes. Executive functioning is a crucial cognitive concept involved in all purposeful behaviour including arousal, attention control and the formation of an action plan in order to complete a task. When explaining it to parents they often remark that in many respects it is synonymous with 'common sense' which is quite a good description or explanation. It is therefore essential for complex purposeful behaviour. At a theoretical level the interrelationship between short term memory, attention, working memory and the central executive was originally proposed in the Baddeley and Hitch (1974) model. The more complex model by Shallice *et al* (1989) can, with a little simplification, prove a useful model to explain some of the problems that are commonly seen in children who have executive functioning disorders. Often parents and teachers can be perplexed by the seemingly intelligent child who acts as though they lack all common sense. In recent years great interest has been directed towards the relationship between frontal lobe functioning and some crucial and wide-ranging developmental disorders including Attention Deficit Disorder (ADD) and the spectrum of Autistic Disorders. The implication of such frontal lobe disorders and functional effects has been extensively explored by Pennington and Oznoff (1996) in their comprehensive review of the subject.

The term 'executive functioning' is therefore used to describe the ability to generate or hypothesise and maintain the appropriate solving set for the attainment of a future goal.

It can be quite separate from other areas in intellectual development such as perception, and many aspects of language and memory. It does, however, overlap with other areas, including attention reasoning and problem-solving. The typical lists used to describe executive functioning include set-shifting and set maintenance, interference control, inhibition, integration of thought across space and time, planning, and working memory. These skills therefore describe a complex range of higher-order cognitive skills which are crucial to independent living.

The sorts of deficits that can occur in adults who have sustained frontal lobe damage have been recognized and reported on by Stuss and Benson (1984) and also assessed (Malloy and Richardson 1994). However, less attention has been paid to the problems associated with such damage in children because this is an aspect of the normal developmental patterns and variance observed in children, and partly because of the educational settings in which they are placed. A young child is not expected to organize himself or plan and execute complex tasks. He is, by virtue of being in a school or a family, structured and focused in much of his day-to-day living. Many of the functions that the frontal lobes control may be masked at a given age. However, some aspects of frontal-lobe functioning can become increasingly apparent as the child gets older (Diamond 1991). Difficulties in attentional control can be less evident and less crucial early in the child's life. Equally, in the more structured primary school environment, the ability to plan and organize is not so crucial in contrast to when the child transfers to secondary school. One pattern that we frequently face is the child who has become overly friendly and disinhibited, with his general social behaviour resembling that of a much younger child, which consequently puts him at considerable risk and causes great anxiety to his parents. Alternatively the child may be over-impulsive, disinhibited, and aggressive in his behaviour, causing frequent disruptions both to home and school life. Rigidity in thinking produces a child who has major difficulties coping with any changes in his environment. Sometimes these children can find life tolerable at primary school, but the transfer to secondary school is usually met with increasing difficulties as they have problems with switching from one set of tasks to another, and having to move from one lesson to another (possibly up to nine times a day) which can frequently prove just too much for them. Passler *et al* (1985) concluded that the development of executive functioning in children occurs in a multi-stage process. Although as yet there is no established, comprehensive list of assessment techniques that can be used for children, one assessment battery of tests has recently been developed for adults (Wilson *et al* 1996).

The rehabilitation of children with frontal-lobe injuries and dysfunction is generally difficult. To some extent, it is possible to focus on areas of specific skills, e.g. children with attentional difficulties can be helped with some intensive tuition and attention-training. It is also possible to encourage a degree of internal control using verbal mediation techniques. Similarly, some problem-solving behaviours can be helped using a 'talking through' approach, having the child verbalize as he works through a problem. In the same way, with a developing child it is possible to teach alternative strategies and through a combination of modelling and guiding, more appropriate codes of behaviour can be encouraged. In the middle and later adolescent years these children can frequently have difficulties at school, not because of the educational demands being placed upon them, but the social demands of their peer group. Other possibly vulnerable children can sense a child who has some of these higher order reasoning difficulties and they can tease or 'set them up'. Therefore the support for many children who have suffered frontal-lobe injuries requires a restructuring of the child's environment. This means a readjustment of parental expectations and demands, which may include an alteration in the organization of the school day and the type of lifestyle that the parents (and family) may have previously led. The child may have to readjust from living within an active, outgoing family to one that follows more structured and solitary pursuits. Similarly, the school environment may have to be modified, in that the child may require individual support or assistance or may need transfer to a special school; however, such a transfer may itself be difficult and necessitate major readjustments.

Problems associated with frontal lobe damage are often complex and on first sight can be confusing and mistaken as signs of emotional disturbance or naughtiness.

Whereas the range of social difficulties can be found using a checklist such as the Vineland Social Adaptation Scales (Sparrow *et al* 1984). These are a descriptive series of statements which refer to normal behavioural competencies and do not identify the underlying neurological deficit. Similarly, IQ measurements are generally not sensitive in picking up such deficits and we see many children who have sustained significant frontal-lobe damage perform competently on conventional intelligence tests. There are however a range of specific tests which are more sensitive to frontal lobe dysfunction, such as the Controlled Verbal Fluency Tests, Wisconsin Card Sort, and Trail-Making Tests. Some of these are interesting in that they make some measure of the child's ability to generate an hypothesis and adapt to a changing situation, i.e. to learn from experience.

Often, children with acute brain injuries do not generalize from the rules of interpersonal behaviour into actual social interchanges. The children appear to be quite concerned about their social relationships and they are often apologetic after making the mistake, and yet they continually repeat the same behaviours and mistakes. These can often be simple aspects of normal social rules , including for instance, remembering to say 'pardon' or 'please' without prompting and following the general school rules. Equally, more subtle problems such as keeping secrets or knowing who and when to tell, may severely affect social relationships. Similarly, exercising self-control by not asking embarrassing or inappropriate questions is crucial if the child is to cope within the social context of a school environment.

To be able to cope socially at a competent level with his peer group, a child must possess the insight and have the ability to read the subtleties in communication such as body language, facial expression, tone of voice, etc. The child who has experienced a brain injury often lacks these skills as well as the ability to process the information and respond within a reasonable time span. He therefore may either not interact, or if he does interact, his approach and behaviour may be inappropriate. He may want to dominate the conversation or does not know when to complete it. As a result, other children may have difficulties understanding his intentions and may misinterpret his behaviour and also his abilities.

REHABILITATION OF SOCIAL COMPETENCE

The child who has frontal lobe dysfunction and is displaying behavioural deficit in the area of executive functioning will ususally benefit from a very structured teaching approach that is based on behavioural methods (Landrus and Mesibox 1994), These make the rules and expectations of classroom behaviour very clear and manage the behaviours in a systematic manner. They do appear to be very effective in helping the child fit into a normal classroom setting. Whereas many schools have behavioural management policies they often rely on the 'normal' child's ability to reason. More systematic packages such as the Assertive Discipline System (Canter and Canter 1976) do appear to be more effective with the child who has had a brain injury as they are much more explicit in their expectations of acceptable behaviours. Whereas this may contain the child's behaviour in a structured setting the child with a brain injury may need some specific social skills retraining. To some extent they can be taught some basic strategies to help them cope with day-to-day living. They can be taught sets of social rules which can then be reinforced and overlearned to the point that they become drilled responses, e.g. stop, look, listen – stop at the kerb, look left, look right, look left again, before crossing. Look outside, check the weather– is it raining? What do I need to wear? etc. These sorts of tasks and exercises are often carried out with younger children, but may only be taught on a casual basis.

Similarly, social behaviour can be taught and children can be given some cues to help them cope, including 'Do not talk to strangers'; 'Do not take sweets from someone that you do not know'; 'Wait for someone else to answer your question before repeating yourself'. Constructive activities such as simple board games can help in coaching the child to develop turn-taking tasks. This can be used as a very positive teaching exercise to encourage him to cooperate in a positive manner with other children. From simple board games the exercise can be further developed, including more children and also more active exercises such as kicking and catching balls and simple team games. Again, the process is to be taught primarily as specific teaching rather than as a physical exercise.

Impulsivity and lack of self-control can be helped by using a cognitive behavioural-modification technique. This basically teaches the child to monitor his own behaviour more effectively and gives him some sort of awareness and self-instruction. The programme is a relatively simple one to operate and usually starts off with some direct modelling of the difficult behaviour. This can be with the use of video material or by means of a teacher or therapist working with the child. The child then imitates the behaviour and through a process of self-instruction using a normal level of voice, he talks himself through a more appropriate strategy. This process is gradually reduced and the child then encouraged to monitor his behaviour by sub-vocalizing the relevant instructions. The child can be encouraged to count to 10 before responding. It is also helpful if he is taught a degree of self-awareness in that if he can feel himself becoming over-aroused and over-excitable he can use alternative strategies including taking himself off to a quiet corner, counting to 10 or more before responding, or taking a deep breath, etc. Some attempts have been made to develop a total package that can be used to teach adolescents a wide range of the necessary social skills that we usually envisage as coming naturally rather than being taught. (Spence 1995). As yet, it is difficult to fully evaluate the value of such a package for brain-injured children, but it does provide a useful source of appropriate teaching ideas and suggestions.

ATTENTION AND POOR CONCENTRATION

Children who have sustained a brain injury frequently have significant difficulties in controlling their attention (Barkley 1996) and they can some-times become overactive. Often they are able to concentrate on activities of their choosing, but have problems when the activity is chosen for them. Unfortunately the term concentration and attention tends to make one focus on the behavioural aspects of the child's problem, (including restlessness), leading to possible disruptiveness rather than a recognition of possible underlying cognitive deficits. The fact that many of these children can attend to self selected tasks can support the opinion that the problem is behavioural. For such children the difficulties more commonly occur when they are asked to switch from one activity to another (divided attention) or sustain their concentration on a given task (sustained attention). A very useful overview of the neuropsychology model of attention is to found in Cooley and Morris (1990) with some detailed discussion of the whole attentional system and different terms that used. Children who have such difficulties appear distractable, impulsive and they can become over-aroused extremely ea-sily. In this situation, they lose self-control and become overexcitable, which can cause behavioural problems with other children. If not recognized and addressed, these problems can result in increasing educational failure and further behavioural problems. It is easy to see how such children can rapidly be labelled as being 'naughty' or having ' behaviour problems ' and the matter seen as a primarily disciplinary rather than a cognitive difficulty.

This pattern of difficulty appears to occur in many of the children who sustain some damage to the frontal areas, although it has to be stated that the precise localization of the attentional processes has proved difficult to determine (Foster *et al* 1994). Medication, e.g. (methyphenidate or Ritalin), may be of use in combination with behavioural methods and some degree of environmental manipulation. It is our experience that this combination of medication and management can be of tremendous benefit to a number of these children, following traumatic brain injuries. The increased awareness of children who have attentional difficulties arising from a developmental disorder has received a great deal of publicity in recent years and has led to the British Psychological Society (1996) establishing a working party to look at the management of such children.

An excellent source book containing detailed teaching examples and management techniques to be found in Clare (1991).

ORGANIZATIONAL DIFFICULTIES

Some brain injured children appear to be very disorganized in their everyday behaviour. They have difficulty in planning and carrying out a single activity or carrying out a series of activities in the correct order. They may forget the order of the day and could well be found looking rather lost and not knowing where they should be, and when. Some of these difficulties can also be seen in the classroom where they may demonstrate difficulties in organizing their thoughts in both oral and written language. This can arise because, despite possessing the necessary vocabulary and basic concepts, they are disorganized in their processing. They may ramble on without ever getting to the point, or they may have difficulty in ordering the information involved into a meaningful and sequential pattern.

Organizational skills are the one aspect of cognition that becomes more crucial as the child gets older. These skills are essential in many aspects of everyday living and also in being able to learn effectively. Again, many of these difficulties do not appear so obvious within an infant or even lower junior school, but as the child progresses through school the ability to organize the information for himself becomes more and more relevant. He may know what he wants to say or write but he is unable to organize it into a meaningful, structured, and coherent pattern. Similarly, he may know what tasks or projects he wants to carry out but he does not know how to start to address the task.

A child's organizational skills are dependent upon the conceptual structure that the child is able to place upon the task and this to an extent, depends upon his long term memory and learning style. The degree of organization can depend upon the previous learning sets the child has acquired. It therefore follows that organization is an active process that a child carries out whilst learning new information. The better he is able to organize then the more efficient the long term retrieval. Organization therefore is a complex activity involving the entire cognitive system, including an efficient awareness of the environment, the ability to isolate, to identify the relevant aspects from the irrelevant ones, and to form new associations. It is therefore necessary that the child evaluates his own performance and readjusts his organizational skills. Such organizational skills are very rarely taught in a precise, detailed manner although some attempt has been made to address this issue, e.g. the Somerset Thinking Skills or through the work by Feurenstien (Feurenstien and Hoffman 1980). Whereas these involve quite detailed programmes, some of their essential elements provide useful sources for information, as well as a basic check-list of tasks for the child to go through in carrying out any problem-solving exercise.

The child who has such difficulties can often be helped with appropriate problem solving strategies. There is a clear need for him to fully define the problem that is to be solved. Frequently, a brain-injured child will start to solve the problem at a very superficial level; there is therefore the need for him to read the problem several times or to encourage him to ask the relevant questions in order that he is fully aware of the task to be completed. The child should then be encouraged to go through a procedure of trying to plan and execute the task. Firstly, he can consider what information is required. A simple check-list for planning and organizing tasks is a useful starting point. He will need to firstly identify and define the problem (i.e. 'What is the problem?'), in which the child is taught not to react impulsively but to think through about the question being asked and what information is going to be required. He can then be encouraged to carry out a 'brain storming' session in which he just jots down one or two simple words about all that he currently knows about the subject. A strategy should then be encouraged for preparing the information, i.e. has he seen a similar problem before, is there anything from previous learning or previous tasks that he can use or adapt in the present situation? He should then be shown how the material can be grouped into some logical order and how it should be best presented in answering the question. The next step is to teach him to think through the problem without first tackling it and to consider what options are available or to think through several different solutions. He should be encouraged to transfer and generalize how the problem-solving approach can be used in other contexts and what lessons can be learnt from the present activities. He can be shown what rules may apply or how a rule could be generated and therefore develop a method of helping him predict how to approach similar problems in the future.

If the child is very young he may understandably have difficulties formulating and understanding the sequence of events. He can be helped to develop these strategies using the following format:

- Structure activities for him. Limit the number of steps in each activity and note them down for the child. At some point the child might find it helpful to have a list of the activities which he has to complete. These could range from what he has to do when he gets up in the morning in order to get ready for school, to the various tasks required during a lesson
- Make sure the child understands what he has to do and, if necessary, make him repeat the tasks back to you.
- Encourage the child to talk himself through some activities as a method of self-monitoring
- Do not assume that the child will remember to do something by himself ; he will frequently need reminding
- Try not to suddenly hurry or rush the child to complete a task because he will be sure to forget something. If a task is to be completed in a given time, make this clear from the start and remind him at regular intervals
- It must be assumed that the child will forget things, e.g. to take his reading book home and to bring it back to school. A selective check is therefore needed just before the child leaves school
- A home/school book, in which messages can be passed between parents and teachers, is a good idea. However, this is sure to be lost unless the child is drilled into putting it somewhere in his bag. If the bag has a special pocket, it is a good idea to put the book in there
- A daily timetable is an invaluable aid to help the child order his daily life. The timetable must include more than just what goes on in school and should include activities from when he gets up in the morning. For older children, two timetables, one for home and another for school, will be required.

For those young children who have very significant difficulties understanding the order of the day and organizing everyday tasks a symbol chart can prove a very useful prompt. The symbols can be easily drawn and different charts can be made for different days of the week thereby helping the child be prepared for changes, as well as following the more mundane routines of everyday life.

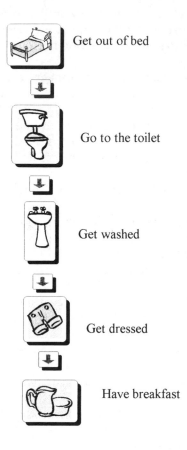

Get out of bed

Go to the toilet

Get washed

Get dressed

Have breakfast

MEMORY

Impairment of memory functioning is one of the most common sequelae of a brain injury and the implications for children is both cumulative and pervasive. Children are in the most active stage of acquiring knowledge and developing skills in every domain. For these reasons any impairment of memory puts them at a considerable disadvantage when compared with their peers. In recent years there have been a number of reports looking at the effects that head injury has on memory functioning. Parallel with this is the development of neuropsychological models of memory functioning, and in particular the work of Bradley (1993) provides an excellent and entertaining overview. However, the serious implications of memory impairment can prove a frightening experience to anyone who has lost their car keys. For a child who has gone through the experience of a hospital admission and disruption to normal life, it can be terrifying. The implications such memory impairment can have on family and academic progress is apparent and well-described by Rivara *et al* (1992). Whereas brain injuries can cause a range of cognitive deficits, possibly one of the most frequently observed in children who have sustained severe head injuries in middle to late childhood, is that of persisting memory disturbance (Prigatano *et al* 1993).

Memory training is therefore an important part of any rehabilitation programme and attempts must be made to teach some basic strategies which have been found relevant in improving memory. However, the term 'memory' is rather oversimplistic because there are a number of different memory functions, each of which can be affected to a lesser or greater extent. In addition, memory deficit may also be caused by problems in attention (concentration) and the processing of information.

Although there have been a number of different concepts of memory and different types of memory which have been described by different authors, (Squire 1987), they tend to share the common idea that memory can be divided into a number of different processes. At a basic functional level it can be divided up into short-term memory (for auditory memory and visual memory) longer-term memory, and working memory.

Short term memory

When considering memory deficits, we find that one of the most common problems encountered relates to the child's short-term memory; that is, his ability to recall information immediately as in repeating back telephone numbers. These sorts of memory problems can commonly show themselves in the child's understanding of language. These children may appear perplexed at times and sometimes wonder why they are being told off when they have done what they think they have been told to do. This can happen if their auditory memory is impaired. They may only respond to the first piece of information in a sentence and not to others. For example, the sentence 'Will you get your games kit ready when you have completed your maths' may be interpreted by the child as 'Get your games kit ready'. These children have significant difficulties when it comes to remembering paragraphs or discussions and only certain key elements of the talk or lesson will be remembered. Sometimes teaching the child visualization techniques or associative techniques (as is often taught to dyslexic children) can give them some useful strategies to support their weak memory.

Children can also have difficulties with visual retention. This typically shows itself in the child not being able to readily recall common words when reading or they may have difficulties copying from the blackboard. It is important that the child has the confidence to be able to ask for information to be repeated or to be shown again. Further techniques aimed at supporting his visual memory can be provided with the use of verbalization; that is, interpreting the diagram verbally in order to provide prompts or cues. In many classroom situations these children can be helped considerably by being given prepared diagrams or partly-completed diagrams rather than being expected to draw them from memory.

Working memory

This is the term used for the ability to hold and manipulate information in immediate consciousness. In computer terms it is sometimes easier to understand as the 'RAM'. It is essential for general problem-solving. The problem can easily be seen in mental arithmetic when the child is given a simple problem such as 'If I bought four bottles of lemonade at 22 pence a bottle, how much change should I expect from £1?'. The child frequently asks for the question to be repeated and is unsure as to what mathematical processes are involved. In these cases, the child can usually complete the problem if the problem is written down as a sum. The child's difficulty can also be observed in reading where he has difficulties with reading comprehension, especially if the answer is not immediately apparent from the text.

In general conversation, the child's stories or even jokes end up as a jumble and sometimes the punchline is given before it is due. These sorts of difficulties cause problems with both social functioning and learning. The previous section on organization gives some ideas as to how to help these children, but as a general rule they have to learn to prepare their thoughts before they speak. This can be done either purely in their head, or they can be told to use a pencil and paper and rather than write down the whole story, they can learn to use key words to help them structure their thoughts more appropriately.

Long term memory

Occasionally, children can acquire very significant functional memory diffi-culties. They wake each morning and can forget what is to happen next, what they need, where they are going, and what day it is. When they go some-where unfamiliar, [or sometimes it can even happen in places that are familiar,] they can find themselves disorientated and forget the way back. In these cases, the development of a simple memory book can be extremely supportive. This consists of a personal book, with the first page comprising a diary sheet with an outline of the main events of the day. Following that is a list of items that would be required and a sequence in which the various activities need to be completed. Timetables should always be included and it is important that the timetable is more detailed than just providing a basic word for a class lesson, e.g. the timetable should also include space for items or material that would be required for each lesson. A number of basic formats are available which can be altered week by week as the requirements at school change. The child can then be encouraged to rely on the book as being the first item to look at, at the start of the day. It is usually left at the side of the bed where it can be examined on waking and also used as the last prompt in the evening to give the child a reminder as to what he may need the next day; it can also serve as a final account for anything that he was able to recall during the day that may have been relevant.

One of the most common methods of aiding memory is, of course, a planned system of revision, and yet it is interesting how little this technique is actually used. Whereas we have all tried to revise the night before that important examination, this is a very inefficient method and a planned revision programme would be more efficient. If long term memory continues to be a problem, the teaching of strategies will be necessary. Diaries may already have been introduced but charts may be vital to put down the day's events in order that activities are not missed. We use weekly charts, with Saturday and Sunday marked differently, so that it is easier for the child to follow. A Filofax may be more appropriate for older children and calendars, clocks, lists, etc. may need to be heavily relied upon. Other external strategies may also be used, e.g., putting a letter near the front door so that it is not forgotten. Internal strategies such as mnemonics may also be a help. These strategies may need to be employed for some time, even indefinitely.

EDUCATIONAL ATTAINMENTS

The educational attainments of any child who has had a significant brain injury and has spent some time in hospital as an inpatient, can be adversely affected in the short term despite the efforts of the Hospital Teaching Services. Fortunately such delays can usually be made up in a short period once the child's life is back to normal. Specific literacy difficulties arising from a brain injury can be complex and in some cases quite unusual such as, the neglect of a part of a word, or difficulty in recognising letters in combination but not in isolation, or even the misreading of words, substituting the actual word with one that has a similar meaning. Whereas these difficulties are well documented in the literature relating to adult acquired conditions (Coltheart 1981), they tend not to be seen so readily or in such a disctinct form in children. This does not mean that the children do not exhibit specific weaknesses but rather may appear to partially compensate quite quickly although they may always have an underlying weakness which is evident on testing. Whereas it is quite apparent from the literature relating to children's head injuries that their academic skills can be quite adversely affected, it is sometimes difficult to fully attribute any reading disability directly to the head injury given a lack of pre-accident skills; and problems may already have been evident before the injury (Shaffer *et al.* (1980)).

To further complicate the matter we see some children make a reasonable recovery and regain their pre-accident level of reading, only for them to then plateau as the child's ability to learn new material and higher order tasks is impaired. Fortunately, the recognition of the specific learning difficulties (ie. dyslexia) that children can manifest, has been well described in recent years (Pumfrey and Reason 1991). With the wider recognition of dyslexia has been the development of specific remedial programmes and specialist courses for teachers. Although an acquired dyslexia is not always the same as one that is developmental in origin, the techniques that can be used are in many cases similar. Most of the programmes are based on a multi-sensory structured teaching approach which is usually quite relevant and applicable to the brain injured child. The programme will most probably need some modification, taking into account the child's particular pattern of strengths and weaknesses. Sometimes such an intensive programme may not be required because the child's difficulties may arise out of a perceptual, attentional or memory deficit which may be addressed in their own right or in combination with a specific remedial programme.

It is important that we do not assume that just because the child can read the material fluently he can also understand it. The brain-injured child may recover some, if not all of his previous reading skills, but he may experience difficulties developing these skills further. Sometimes his actual reading accuracy may appear within the normal range, but he may demonstrate significant difficulties in understanding what he has read. If this is the problem, encourage the child to read and re-read the text and then underline key points in it to aid his comprehension. Because of the potential problems with comprehension, it is sometimes helpful to prepare the child with the material to be read. This can be done by using either paired reading or relaxed reading strategies, e.g. reading the material to the child at least once before he reads it himself.

Recorded literacy

Writing fluently is a complex multi-tasking operation which involves a number of different processes. To work efficiently and smoothly many of the sub-skills have to be learnt to the point at which they become automatic – a bit like driving a car. If the child has to concentrate on letter formation or spelling then it follows that they cannot attend to content, grammar, or punctuation.

Brain injury can frequently result in significant problems in retrieving information. Spelling and writing are examples where there must be a swift, accurate interpretation and transcription of thoughts onto paper, and this may be impaired. The brain-injured child may be left with some motor coordination or organizational difficulties and a well-structured handwriting scheme is essential to provide him with a mental framework within which to operate.

The child may have difficulties acquiring basic spelling skills. This is usually the case when the brain injury has occurred in young children who had not developed their spelling skills at the time of the injury. It has long been recognized that for children with any sort of specific learning difficulty, a multi-sensory learning approach has much to offer, and this is certainly the case for the brain-injured child. This simply means that we try to involve as many senses as possible in the learning situation. Again, a well-thought-out scheme such as one of those used for dyslexic pupils can be very helpful, and it helps to organize the need for regular and planned revision.

Organization of written work

Whereas the problems of organizational skills have been discussed with regards to behaviour, a child may have problems organizing his thoughts when writing stories or writing up projects. Just as his personal behaviour needs organizing, so does his ability to express himself on paper. He will benefit from some help in drafting and in essay-planning techniques. Some discussions may have already taken place over this, but these children can be helped by more formal and structured approaches. A simple planning sheet can be used which may help them in many situations.

Whenever possible, the child should be given work that includes a closed procedure, e.g. sentence completion, a passage with blanks to fill in, or a selection of words to place in the correct order. Fortunately, the idea of providing children with some structure to aid their writing appears to be in the process of returning and the use of writing frames appears to be becoming more generally used.

Mathematics

Specific disorders of mathematical skills have never received the attention that dyslexia has until comparatively recently, despite the fact that developmental dyscalculia is considered to be a relatively common disorder. There is therefore a general lack of expertise and material to draw upon. However this is an area which is now receiving increasing attention and there is a greater awareness of the specific deficits that children can suffer in their development of numeracy skills. Temple (1989 and 1991) decribes some of the specifc deficits that can occur in mathematical processing and clearly there are a number of aspects of mathematics with which the brain injured child may experience difficulties including conceptual, short term memory, perceptual and spatial deficits.

There are a number of children who may find it hard to conceptualise numbers and deal with them in an abstract manner. At this stage the child will need plenty of practical experience in working with materials and he needs to be encouraged to continue to use such material when computing. The use of language as a mediating tool is one way of helping the child develop the concept. A recent text by Nunes and Bryant (1996) offers more detailed insight into such processes.

When short term memory is impaired, the child may find difficulty in remembering all of a question. He can make frequent and silly mistakes because of this problem and not because of errors in computation. If this is thought to be the problem it is helpful to get him into the habit of writing down the question in note form before he attempts to carry out any computation. In general we find that many of the approaches used with dyslexic children are also a useful source of ideas for the brain injured child, (Miles and Miles 1992).

Children who have spatial or perceptual deficits may be capable of carrying out the underlying mathematical calculations and errors occur most frequently when figures are not aligned correctly before computation. The actual process of copying a set of figures from a board or even a text book to their exercise book increases the chance of producing numerous errors. Problems such as these are often solved quite easily by providing the child with some structure and squared paper is of course one of the easiest methods especially with the traditional prompts (Hundreds, Tens and Units) at the top of columns. Prepared worksheets are another obvious solution and certainly remove the opportunity for errors to occur in the initial copying down stage.

Sometimes the child may have difficulties remembering sequences and it is apparent that he will have difficulty in remembering instructions and processes involved in problem solving. Care should be taken to ensure that such processes are broken down into manageable steps. These should be well laid out and graphically illustrated, possibly using coloured felt tip pens to high-light or emphasise the various steps.

To function competently in maths a number of sub-skills and processes need to be taught to a level whereby they are implicitly known. The child who has a brain injury may have great difficulty with such rote learning tasks, as might be demonstrated in his difficulty in remembering multiplication tables.

The child will need a lot of repetition in order that he can acquire these to a proficient and automatic level.

Fatigue

It must be emphasized that one of the main problems facing the brain-injured child when he returns to his normal school environment is the level of fatigue that many of the children appear to have. It is not uncommon to find the brain-injured child being reported as going to sleep as soon as he comes home from school, or even during school. Frequently, it is difficult for him to sustain any level of effort and application for a normal school day, and part-time placement may be initially required. Even when he is able to cope with a full day in school he can often find coping with homework extremely difficult, and of course, any form of social life after school is rapidly eroded or even abandoned due to tiredness. In such cases it is important to try to work with the child and parents in order that he can pace himself and come to realistic expectations and goals. It may be very useful for the child to develop a schedule which outlines aims and objectives which need to be completed within the coming weeks. It is clearly important that dedicated periods for relaxation, leisure, or quality-of-life experiences are incorporated into this schedule, as a failure to do so may prove counter productive and frustrating, and he may continue to try and achieve what is largely unachievable.

RETURN TO MAINSTREAM SCHOOL

As the child progresses through the rehabilitation process, the return to mainstream becomes ever apparent. Sometimes this is an easy procedure, but with increasing demands within the mainstream setting, a positive link between hospital school and home school is essential to this end. There is a DFE NHS Executive, Department of Health Joint Circular requesting such collaboration. At Alder Hey, a key member of the head-injury rehabilitation team (HIRT) is the link teacher, who becomes familiar with the child whilst he is an in patient and attending the hospital school, and therefore can act as a stable, familiar figure.

A teacher who can link in with the child's own school is crucial in smoothing the hand-over from the hospital to his previous school. Once the child is well enough to restart his own school, he may feel that he has fully recovered. He will probably be unaware of the extent to which the brain injury may have affected him and the changes in personality and cognitive functioning that could possibly have taken place. It may therefore come as something of a shock to him when he realizes that he may not find his school-work as easy as he did previously. It is distinctly possible that he will be unable to keep up with his peer group, which can cause old friendships to break up, and he may experience difficulties forming new ones. Subtle changes in his learning or personality may have taken place; other children may slowly become aware of this, and it may unsettle him. He may make new friendships with less mature children, which can exaggerate episodes of silly behaviour. The return to school is therefore not necessarily an easy or straightforward one.

In order to prepare the way for the child, regular contact is maintained with his previous school prior to reintegration. Usually this is achieved by reporting his progress in the rehabilitation programme and giving an outline of his individual education programme (IEP). A reintegration programme is devised; initially, one session or one day in the mainstream, returning to the hospital school for the remainder of the week, increasing as and when appropriate. The programme is carefully monitored and can be modified at any time. On completion of the programme, contact is kept and the child is followed up for as long as is necessary. This period of gradual and progressive integration also helps to sensitize the receiving school that the child's needs have to be looked at in terms other than academic progress and basic educational attainments. If the child has any specific difficulties these are made known to the special-needs coordinator within the mainstream school, who is the person who must, under the terms of the 1993 Education Act, be fully familiar with the specific needs of individual children. In addition, it is equally important that the child's class-teacher is fully aware of any difficulties.

A child with a brain injury takes time to re-establish himself within the classroom group. It may have been only a matter of weeks that the child has been absent, or alternatively, it may have been many months. The child may be returning to a classroom environment in which friendship groups have altered considerably since he was there. New friendships will have to be established and overtures made to old friends who may now have formed new friendships themselves. The child will find that much work will have been completed since he was last in school. He will therefore be unfamiliar with much of it . His ability to compete with other children will have been impaired, and even keeping up with some of the routine classroom duties will prove difficult. He is also likely to fatigue quickly; therefore maintaining the pace throughout the duration of the whole school day will prove extremely difficult, if not impossible, at least in the early stages.

Even when all the best preparations are made, things can go wrong for a number of reasons, as explained by one of our children.

Letter written by Anthony

I understand that I had an accident on the 16th February 1995. I cannot remember the actual accident. In fact, I can't remember when it happened. All I can remember is what other people have told me about it.

My friend came down to see me because I was not very well and we decided to walk over to Asda to buy something; my mum said it was for her. As we crossed the road I was told that there were parked cars. My brother offered to go with me as we had finished tea, but we didn't want to wait for him. On the way back my friend offered me a sweet, but he told me that I didn't take it because I said I wasn't feeling very well. Well, that is the last thing I can remember.

I woke up on Ward D3 at Alder Hey. I was told that I was taken to Fazakerley Hospital initially, and then I was transferred to the intensive care unit at Alder Hey. As well as the head injury I had fractures around my waist, and when I woke up I couldn't talk properly, I couldn't walk, and my hands and arms didn't seem to work properly. I can remember feeling very frightened, but people kept saying 'not to worry', and telling me to 'relax'.

Well, I stayed in Alder Hey for several weeks. While I was on the ward people came and I can remember doing something called speech therapy, physiotherapy, and occupational therapy. I can't remember very much now what they did, but they did make me do things. I can remember feeling very tired and I didn't always want to work, but they said I had to. When I was well enough, I started to go down to the hospital school. I felt better there because it seemed more like normal life. The work seemed easy and if I had any problems there was always someone to turn to.

When I left the hospital and started to sleep at home, I carried on coming into the hospital school for quite a while. They said it was so I could get better and catch up with my work. I stayed in the hospital school for about four months and then there were some meetings with teachers from my old school. They said that they would help me and they arranged for me to gradually go back to school. It was all right at first, everyone was very kind and they helped me a lot but I soon found the work was too hard for me. There were lots of other children in the classes and if I didn't know what I was doing no one seemed to help. It was very difficult to get the teacher to come over to me. I became more and more frustrated and felt like 'lashing out at someone'. It was no one's fault. There were just too many children in the class. I also had problems because I sometimes got lost. I used to lose my timetable and then I would have to go to the office and it would take ages to try to find out where I should be.

When I left the hospital school I asked if someone could look after me and help me from class to class. That worked at first but the person soon lost interest, and anyway, sometimes we were not in the same class and they would rush off and leave me stranded. I started to have days off because I felt I couldn't cope. The days off became more and more as I found it easier to take the day off rather than go into school. I felt far more desperate, I wasn't getting anywhere and I was falling further and further behind with my work.

EXTRA SUPPORT

In almost one third of the children we treat in the HIRT programme, it is not possible for the child to return to his own mainstream school. Under these circumstances, the child may require statementing under the terms of the 1993 Education Act. Many parents find this a frightening and daunting experience since there is the immediate implication that the child may have long-term problems. Fortunately, this may not be the case and it may simply mean that the child needs additional classroom assistance for very practical problems, for example, if he has a tracheostomy or requires assistance with mobility or toileting. Alternatively, it may be that the child has some learning difficulties and needs extra support in class.

The statementing procedure has to be carried out by the child's own local education authority. The criteria for statementing and the provision required varies considerably from authority to authority, and sometimes it is necessary for the parents to have an advocate in order to ensure that the child's needs are fully addressed. The very specific needs of a brain-injured child can be overlooked by an education authority which uses the hard criteria of measured delay in educational attainments as a criteria for statementing. Such simplistic approaches can exclude a child who has subtle deficits that can interfere with the effectiveness of new learning but have possibly left old learning relatively intact. This approach may leave the child in a situation in which he almost stands still (academically) until his level falls well below that of his peers and to the point where his education authority will consider statementing. Fortunately, under the terms of the Education Act there is a requirement for the advice of other professionals to be included and therefore the reports and recommendations from the head-injury-team can be included in the child's statement. However what is really important is to try to ensure that any recommendations are actually formally written into the child's statement. Unfortunately recommendations or levels of support are often written in such general terms that they can become almost meaningless.

On rare occasions following a brain injury it is necessary for the child to attend a special school. The child may have significant learning difficulties or behaviour problems that would render him disadvantaged within a mainstream setting, no matter what level of support was provided. It may be that these children would benefit from a small-group classroom setting in which the presentation of work and the level of tasks can be individually devised. In most circumstances the special school offers a suitable and secure environment for the brain-injured child, but unfortunately, the class teachers will not be fully aware of his needs. By virtue of it's role, most special schools cater for children who have developmental difficulties and not for children who have acquired difficulties. Whereas there is a degree of similarity in the learning processes of both groups, the cognitive deficit of a brain-injured child can be complex, subtle or severe. The difficulties can be much more specific than those usually encountered in children with developmental problems and these differences are not always fully recognized. In addition, the brain injured child may feel ill at ease with children who have grown up with their disability. There is therefore the need for the greater understanding of the very specific needs of the brain injured child throughout the educational system.

REFERENCES

Baddeley, A.D. and Hitch, G. (1974). Working memory, in *The psychology of learning and motivation* (ed. G.A. Bower). Academic Press, New York, 8, 47–89.

Bain A.M., Bailet, L.L., and Moats, L. C. (1991). *Written language disorders: theory into practice*. Taskmaster Ltd, Leicester.

Barkley R. A. (1996). Attention deficit hyperactivity disorder. In *Child psychopathology* (ed. E. J. Marsh and R. A. Barkley). Guildford Publication, New York.

Bawden, H.N., Knights, R.M., and Winogron, H.W. (1985). Speeded-performance head injury in children. *Journal of Clinical Neuropsychology*, 7, 39–54.

Beery, K.E. (1989). *The developmental test of visual motor integration*. Modern Curriculum Press, Cleveland, Toronto.

Blagg, N., Ballinger, M., and Gardner, R. (1989). *Somerset thinking skills*. Blackwell, Oxford.

Bradley, A. (1993). *Your memory : an owner's guide*. Penguin Press, London.

British Psychological Society Report. (1996). *Attention deficit hyperactivity disorder. A psychological response to an evolving concept*. BPS Publication, Leicester.

Borod, J.C. (1992). Interhemispheric and intrahemispheric control of emotion. *Journal of Consulting and Clinical Psychology*, 60, 339–48.

Brooks, N. (1984). Cognitive deficits after head injury. In *Closed head injury: psychosocial, social and family consequences* (ed. N. Brooks), pp. 4473 Oxford Community Press, Oxford.

Buzan, T. (1995). *Use your head*. BBC, London

Canter, L. and Canter, M. (1976). *Assertive discipline*. Lee Canter Associates, santa Monica.

Caramazza, A. (1990). *Cognitive neuropsychology and neurolinguistics*. Lawrence Erlbaum, London.

Clare, B.J. (1991). *Sourcebook for children with attention deficit disorder*. Communication Skill Builders, Wimslow Press, Oxon.

Code of Practice on Identification and Assessment of Special Educational Needs (1994). Central Office of Information.

Coltheart, M. (1981). Disorders of reading and their implications for models of normal reading, *Visible Language*, 15, 245–86.

Cooley, E.L. and Morris, R.D, (1990). Attention in children: a neuropsychologically based model for assessment. *Developmental Neuropsychology*, 6, 239–74.

Cruickshank, W.M., Bentzen., F.A., Ratzeborgh, F.H., and Tannhauser, M.T. (1961). *A teaching method for brain-injured and hyperactive children. A demonstration pilot study.* Syracuse University Press, Syracuse.

Diamond, A. (1991) Neuropsychological insights into the meaning of object concept development. In *The epigenisis of mind: essays on biology and cognition* (ed. S. Carey and R. Gelman). Lawrence Erlbraum Association, Hillsdale.

Elliott, C.D., Murray, D.J. and Pearson, L.S. (1983). *British Abilities Scales*. NFER-Nelson, Berkshire.

Ellis, A.W. and Young, A.W. (1988). *Human cognitive neuropsychology*. Lawrence Erlbaum, London.

Feuerstein, R. and Hoffman, M. B. (1980). *Instrumental enrichment*. Park Press, Baltimore.

Foster, J. K., Eskes, G. A., and Strun, D. T. (1994). The cognitive neuropsychology of attention: a frontal-lobe perspective. *Cognitive Neuropsychology*, 11, 133–47.

Frostig, M. (1966). *The Marianne Frostig Developmental Test of Visual Perception*. Consulting Psychologists Press, Palo Alto, California.

Gardner, M.F. (1982). *Test of Visual Perceptual Skills (non-motor)*. Psychological and Educational Publications, Inc., California.

Golden, C. J. (1981). The Luria-Nebraska children's battery: theory and formulation. In *Neuropsychological assessment and the school age child: issues and procedures*, (ed. G. W. Hynd and J. E. Obryent). Grime and Stratton, New York.

Goswomi, V. and Bryant, P. (1991). *Phonological skills and learning to read*. British Library Cataloguing in Publication Data. BPCC. Wheatons, Exeter.

Grodjinsky, G. M. and Diamond, R. (1992). Frontal-lobe Functioning in boys with ADD. *Developmental Neuropsychology*, 8, 427–45.

Johnson, D.A., Utterley, D., and Wylie, M. (1989). *Children's head injury: who cares?* Taylor and Francis, London, and New York.

Johnson, D.A. (1992). Head-injured children and education: a need for greater delineation and understanding. *British Journal of Educational Psychology*, 62, 404–9.

Kaufman, A.S. (1994). *Intelligence testing with the WISC-111*. John Wiley, New York.

Kelly, T.P., Borrill, H.S., and Maddell, D.L. (1996). Development and assessment of executive function in children. *Child Psychology and Psychiatry Review*, 1, 46–51.

Kolb, K. and Whishaw, I.Q. (1996). *Fundamentals of human neuropsychology*. W.H. Freeman and Co.

Landrus, R.I. and Mesibov, G.B. (1994). *'TEACCH': Structured teaching*. University of North Carolina, Carolina.

Lezak, M.D. (1995). *Neuropsychological Assessment*. Oxford University Press, Oxford.

Lezak, M.D. (1988). IQ. R.I.P. *Journal of Clinical and Experimental Neuropsychology*, 10, 351–61

Luria, A.R. (1976). *The man with a shattered word*. Regnery, Chicago.

Malloy, P.F. and Richardson, D.E. (1994). Assessment of fronta-lobe functions. *Journal of Neuropsychiatry*, 6, 399–410.

Mesulam, M. (1986). Frontal cortex and behaviour neurology. *Annals of Neurology*, **19**, 4320–5.

Miles, T. R. and Miles, E. (1992). *Dyslexia and mathematics*. Routledge, London and New York.

Milton, S.R., Scaglione, C., Flanagan, T., Cox, J. *et al.* (1991). Functional Evaluation of adolescent students with traumatic brain injury. *Journal of Head Trauma Rehabilitation*, **6**, 35–45.

Nunes, T. and Bryant, P. (1996). *Children doing mathematics*. Blackwell, Oxford.

Oddy, M. (1993) Head injury during childhood. *Neuropsychological Rehabilitation*, **3**, 301–20.

Passler, M.A., Issac, W., and Hynd, G.W. (1985). Neuropsychological development of behaviour attributed to frontal-lobe functioning in children. *Developmental Neuropsychology*, **1**, 349–70.

Pennington, B.F. and Oznoff, S. (1996). Executive functioning and developmental psychopathology. *Journal of Child Psychology and Psychiatry*, **37**, 58–89.

Prigatano, G.P., O'Brien, K.P., and Klonoff, P.S. (1983). Neuropsychological rehabilitation of young adults who suffer brain injury in childhood: clinical observations. *Neuropsychological Rehabilitation*, **3**, 411–21.

Pumfrey, P.D. and Reason, R.R. (1991). *Specific learning difficulties {Dyslexia}*. NFER-Nelson, Berkshire.

Reitan, R. M. (1981). *Effects of age of onset of brain damage on later development*. Presented at Reitan Neuropsychological Workshop, Chicago.

Rivara, J.B., Fay G., Jaffe, K., Polissar, N., Shritleff, H., and Martin, K. (1992) Predictors of family functioning one year following traumatic brain injury in children. *Archives of Physical Medicine and Rehabilitation*, **73**, 899–912.

Schacter, D.L. and Crovity, H.F (1977). Memory function after a closed head injury: a review of quantitative research. *Cortex* . **13**, 150–76.

Shaffer, D., Bijur, P., Chadwick, O. and Rutter, M. (1980). Head injury and later reading disability. *Journal of the American Academy of Child Psychiatry*, **19**, 592–610.

Shallice, T., Burger, P., Schon, F. and Baxter, D. (1989). The origins of utilisation behaviour. *Brain*, **112**, 1587–98.

Sparrow, S., Balla, D., and Cichetti, D.V. (1984). *Vineland adaptive behaviour scales*. American Guidance Service, Inc., Minnesota.

Spence, S. (1995). *Social-skills training with children and adolescents*. NFER-Nelson, Berkshire.

Squire, L.R. (1987). *Memory and brain*. Oxford University Press, New York.

Strauss, E. and Spreen, O. (1991). *A compendium of neuropsychological tests*. Oxford University Press, Oxford.

Stuss, D.T. and Benson, F.D. (1984). Neuropsychological studies of the frontal lobes. *Psychological Bulletin*, **95**, 3–28.

Telygrow C.P. (1987) Management of academic and educational problems in head injury. *Journal of Learning Disabilities*, **20**, 9, 536–45.

Temple, C.M. (1989). The cognitive neuropsychology of the developmental dyscalculias. *Current Psychology of Cognition*, **133**, 351–70.

Temple, C.M. (1991). procedural Dyscalcula and Number fact dyscalculia: Double dissociation in developmental dyscalculia. *Cognitive Neuropsycholgy*, **8**, 155–76.

Tromp, E. and Mulder, T. (1991). Neuropsychological slowness of information processing after a traumatic head injury. *Journal of Clinical and Experimental Neuropsychology*, **13**, 821–30.

Warrington, E.K. and James, M. (1991). *The Visual Object and Space Perception Battery*. Thames Valley Test Company, Bury St Edmunds, Suffolk, England.

Wechsler Intelligence Scale for Children III-UK. (1992). The Psychological Corporation, Harcourt & Brace, London.

Wilson, B.A., Alderman, N., Burgess, P.W., Emslie, H., and Evans, J.J. (1996). *Behavioural assessment of the dysexecutive syndrome*. Thames Valley Test Group, England.

Wrightson, P., McGinn, V., and Gronwall, D. (1995). Mild head injury in preschool children: evidence that can be associated with a persisting cognitive defect. *Journal of Neurology, Neurosurgery, and Psychiatry*, **59**, 375–80.

9

Emotional, behavioural, and social difficulties

Colin Demellweek, Audrey O'Leary, and Tony Baldwin

INTRODUCTION

Although the term 'emotional, behavioural, and social difficulties' is used in this chapter, these problems may also be referred to as being psychosocial, psychiatric, neuropsychiatric, or as reflecting personality or characterological changes. These differences exist since it is possible to view problems from different perspectives. For example, irritability appears to be common following brain injury (BI). This may be considered to be emotional (i.e. feelings of irritation are more intense and frequent), the behavioural consequences of which may interfere with social relationships and, if persistent, be seen as an aspect of the individual's personality or character. Similarly, depression may occur following BI. Again this may be referred to as being emotional or as being psychiatric or neuropsychiatric and would be expected to have behavioural and social consequences. Terms will therefore be used as in the original studies referred to.

Most of the studies referred to in this chapter are of children who have suffered head injuries (HI). It is, however, the injury to the brain which is most important, and emotional, behavioural, and social sequelae appear to be similar when BI is caused by a non-traumatic cerebral insult, including infective, metabolic or hypoxic encephalopathies. The term 'BI ' will therefore be used in this chapter unless reference is made to a particular study of children with HI. Although BI in children is mostly caused by a blow to the head, it is unclear precisely how forceful the blow needs to be to injure the brain. Children with, in particular, mild HI may therefore have no *obvious* brain injury.

TYPES OF EMOTIONAL, BEHAVIOURAL, AND SOCIAL PROBLEMS SEEN AFTER BRAIN INJURY IN CHILDREN

These can be many and varied and include; social disinhibition or acting in socially inappropriate ways, irritability, increased emotionality, reduced judgement and motivation, perseveration, lowered tolerance to frustration, egocentricity seen through insensitivity to others, unawareness of their impact on others, and an increase in demanding behaviour (Lehr 1990). Added to this list can be; impulsivity, fearfulness, anxiety and depression, verbal and physical aggression, discipline problems, sleep disturbance, eating problems (over and undereating), overactivity, a tendancy to make facile jokes, and gullibility (Deaton and Waaland 1994). Many of the emotional and behavioural problems seen after BI are similar to those that occur in the general population, the exception being marked socially disinhibited behaviour such as the making of very personal remarks (Brown *et al*. 1981). The cause of a particular problem may, however, be different following BI. For example, temper outbursts may be more related to difficulties with self-control and frequent experience of frustration whilst there may also be greater felt and expressed remorse after the outburst.

FREQUENCY OF BEHAVIOURAL, EMOTIONAL, AND SOCIAL PROBLEMS

Research into the likelihood of children developing emotional and behavioural problems following a BI has produced somewhat mixed results. An early study (Brown *et al*, 1981) compared children who had suffered a mild or severe HI with controls who had suffered orthopaedic injuries. Pre-morbidly (i.e. prior to the injury), approximately 11% of the controls had a psychiatric disorder, rising to 22% at 1 year and 28% at just over 2 years post-injury. In the severely head-injured group, 21% of children were found to have a pre-morbid psychiatric disorder, rising to 53% at 1 and 2 years post-injury. In the mildly head injured group 34% of the children had a premorbid psychiatric disorder, falling to 24% at 1 year post-injury and then increasing to 34% at 2 years post-injury. The development of new psychiatric disorders after the injury had been sustained was significantly higher in severely, but not mildly, head-injured children compared to controls. It was also noted that of the 14 severely head-injured children who did not have any pre-morbid abnormality, only 28% had a definite psychiatric disorder at the 1 year follow-up. In contrast, of the 11 children with severe HI who had trivial or dubious psychiatric disorders pre-morbidly, 54% had a definite disorder at 1 year follow-up.

Some studies (which have excluded children with pre-morbid problems) have, however, found an increase in behavioural and emotional problems following mild HI. In one study (Asarnow *et al*, 1991), parents completed a behaviour problem check-list on the head-injured child at least 1 year after the injury had been sustained. In the mild head injured group, 66% had a total behaviour-problem score in the clinical range whereas 72.7% of children with severe HI did so. In another study (Rivara *et al*, 1992), approximately 25% of parents reported that, 1 year following a mild HI, the child was more irritable, had more temper outbursts, and his personality had changed. The reasons for these discrepancies are unclear because studies often differ on a number of variables such as the criteria used to exclude children, the types of assessments carried out, the criteria used to define HI severity, and the time since injury when problems are assessed.

It is well-established that adults commonly report having psychological problems such as anxiety and depression following BI (Morton and Wehman 1995). Only one study (in which children with pre-morbid problems were also excluded), however, appears to have examined children's self-reported adjustment following HI (Andrews *et al*, 1993); in this study, moderately and severely injured children were shown to have significantly lower self-esteem than (uninjured) controls.

CAUSES OF BEHAVIOURAL, EMOTIONAL, AND SOCIAL PROBLEMS

There may be many reasons why a child develops such problems following a BI (Asarnow *et al*, 1991), some of which are outlined in Fig. 9.1. There is, however, a lack of research into this area, particularly with children. Thus, the factors outlined in Fig. 9.1 are based largely on findings with adults with BI, clinical observations drawn from the literature, and personal experience. The formulation outlined must, therefore, be considered provisional. For reasons of clarity, some potential links between the factors outlined in Fig. 9.1 are not shown in the diagram but are referred to in the text. It should also be noted that, first, the causes of particular behaviour problems may change with time. For example, temper tantrums seen shortly after the BI has been sustained may be due to disinhibition. If, however, the tantrums are effective in obtaining rewards, then such behaviour may continue even though the ability for self-inhibition improves. Second, in some cases deficits may be silent for a time following BI. Thus, problems due to executive dysfunction may not be marked until the child becomes of an age when more self-determination is required. Third, children with BI are likely to be exposed to stress not related to the injury, such as the death of a grandparent. Because of the BI, however, they may be less able to deal with such stresses.

Pre-morbid difficulties

Behavioural and emotional problems shown by children, following BI, may, of course, have existed prior to the injury. Indeed, some problems, e.g. excessive risk-taking, attentional difficulties, and clumsiness, may increase

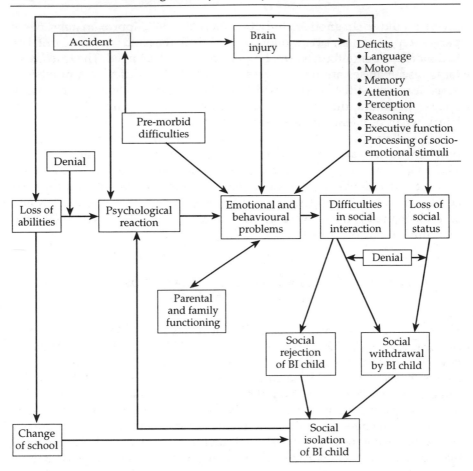

Fig. 9.1 Causes of behavioural, emotional, and social problems following brain injury.

the likelihood of a child being injured. There are, however, discrepancies in the literature concerning the pre-morbid characteristics of children who suffer BI. Thus, an early study (Brown *et al*, 1981) reported that 34.5% of mild HI children had a pre-morbid psychiatric disorder compared to 21.4% of children with a severe HI and 10.7 per cent of controls. A more recent study, (Donders 1992) however, found that only 11% of children referred to an in-patient rehabilitation unit following HI had clinically significant pre-morbid behaviour problems compared to an expected incidence in the general population of 10%. There was, however, a tendency for mildly injured children to have more pre-morbid behaviour problems than severely injured children. Similarly, in a study of children admitted to neurosurgical units (Pelco *et al*, 1992) the mean pre-morbid score on a behaviour problem check-list was not significantly higher than that of children in the community. Between 15 and 20% of the children had clinically significant pre-morbid behaviour problems. Again, the reasons for these discrepancies are unclear, but may be multiple.

Parent and family functioning

It would be expected that any emotional and behavioural problems shown by the child, following BI, would both influence, and be influenced by, parental and family functioning. The general effect of having a child suffer a BI on such functioning is discussed in Chapter 11. In this section, therefore, the emphasis will be on parenting style which is known to have a considerable influence on children's psychosocial development (Berk 1992). Sometimes, parents appear to expect too much of the brain-injured child, which can lead them to accuse him of not trying with consequent effects on his psychological functioning (see Chapter 11). Clinical experience suggests, however, that it is more common for parents to have difficulty in setting and maintaining appropriate limits for brain-injured children. There appears to be two major aspects to this difficulty. Parents do appear to be able to set and maintain firm limits relating to the child's safety, but such limits often seem to be too strict. Limits they set in other areas, however, may be too lax, or, appropriate limits may be set but then abandoned when the child protests.

Overprotection

A number of observers have commented on the tendency of parents to overprotect brain-injured children, for which there is some empirical support. Thus, in one small study of young males aged 14–25 years with severe disabilities following BI, a common complaint was that they were not allowed to take minor risks. In the general population it appears that such overprotection reflects parental anxiety and, in particular, feelings that the world is not a safe place (Thomasgard and Metz 1993). Carers of adult survivors of BI can show heightened levels of anxiety which may continue for a long period of time following the injury, whilst parents' assumptions about invulnerability and that the world is a just place may be affected when their child has a BI (see Chapter 11).

The possible effects of overprotection on children may include overdependency or separation anxiety but is likely to depend on the reaction of the child (Thomasgard and Metz 1993). Young children or children who themselves do not feel safe may accept parental overprotection. Children who have, however, been used to making some safety decisions for themselves and are ready to do so again, may resist being overprotected. The effects of overprotection may also depend on the level of care the child receives. Adults who experienced high levels of both care and protection during their own childhood ('affectionate constraint') are prone to develop hypochondriasis or panic attacks, whereas adults who experienced low care and high protection in childhood ('affectionless control') are prone to depression (Parker 1990).

Overindulgence

After a child has had a BI, inappropriate behaviour may go unchallenged, items the child wants (toys, clothes, food, etc.) may be immediately provided, and rules relating to bedtime etc. may not be enforced if the child protests. This can be seen as overindulgence, which can be defined as excessive gratification of the child coupled with a lack of control (Thomasgard and Metz 1993). There may be two major reasons for such parental behaviour. First, overindulgence in general is thought to be linked to parental feelings of guilt (Thomasgard and Metz 1993), and a number of observers have commented that parents often feel guilty after their child has had a BI. Many parents seem to think, very often without good reason, that they have failed to protect the child. Parents can also feel guilty for being angry with their brain-injured child (Leichtman 1992), thus punishments may be set in anger and then quickly rescinded because of guilt. Second, parents naturally and understandably feel a great deal of sympathy for the injured child. This, together with feelings of guilt, may lead to attempts to compensate the child for the losses he has suffered, materially or in other indulgences. If, as discussed later, the child has lost friends and become more socially isolated following the BI, parents may try to compensate by becoming his friend or playmate. Parents may also do this if they are reluctant to allow the child to play outside or engage in particular activities.

Although such tendencies on the part of parents are understandable, there may well be negative repercussions. Switching between roles as playmate and parent may lead to confusion about parental authority. In addition, if parents are usually available to be playmates the child's motivation to learn to relate to peers may be reduced. Furthermore, the various treats (material or otherwise) the BI child is given can be resented by peers and siblings. Parental overindulgence may serve to promote child dominance within the family (Thomasgard and Metz 1993) which is likely to make the child feel insecure and so possibly seek to challenge other authority figures such as teachers.

Lack of parental confidence

Another reason for parental difficulty in setting and maintaining limits, not linked to safety for the brain-injured child, relates to a lack of parental confidence. Learned helplessness may have developed during the child's stay in hospital and the rehabilitation unit (see Chapter 11), so that parents feel de-skilled when the child returns home. Parents may also be unsure as to what is reasonable to expect from the child, and, in particular, to what extent certain behaviours (e.g. swearing) reflect BI rather than other factors. Even experienced psychotherapists can sometimes find such judgements difficult to make (Judd 1988). Parents understandably, therefore, may tend to err on the side of caution. A thorough neuropsychological assessment can clarify this issue to some extent, but there is always likely to be some uncertainty. For example, testing may indicate that a child has memory problems but cannot determine in every instance whether the child truly forgot something or is using this as an excuse. A lack of parental confidence may result in permissive parenting in which parents avoid asserting their authority. Such a style of parenting tends to result in children who are demanding, immature, have difficulty in controlling their impulses, and are disobedient and explosive if asked to do something they do not wish to do (Berk 1991).

Pre-morbid parenting difficulties

Although it is not shown in Fig. 9.1, it is possible that parenting difficulties, which existed prior to the injury, are linked to any pre-morbid behaviour problems shown by the brain-injured child, and may be heightened following the injury. For example, parents who were abused as children may tend to be overprotective because of beliefs that the world is a dangerous place (Thomasgard and Metz 1993). Such beliefs are likely to be reinforced when a child suffers a BI, thereby increasing the tendency towards overprotection.

Cognitive and other deficits

The cognitive and other deficits which commonly occur following BI can have a considerable impact on the social, emotional, and behavioural functioning of children.

Motor impairment

Adults appear to cope well with motor impairment which can result from BI. Such impairments are, however, more likely to have an effect on children since their social life often involves much more physical activity, in the form of games and sports, than that of adults. In addition, physical ability plays an important part in children's – particularly boys' self-esteem (Berk 1991). Indeed, one young boy who was left with motor impairments, following BI, saw himself as being broken (Judd 1988). The precise effect of acquired motor impairment on the child, however, may depend on a number of factors. For example, a child who is very interested in, and good at, sports may be particularly affected by a motor impairment, following BI.

Language problems

Obvious language problems will clearly affect social interaction. Following a BI, however, a child may be able to talk but not to communicate (Dennis 1991), i.e. social discourse may be affected. The child may have difficulty in knowing the alternative meanings of words in context (e.g. the duck was ready to eat), getting the point of figurative or metaphoric expressions (e.g. she was easily crushed), bridging inferential gaps in interpersonal situations, and describing verbally the apparent intention of others. Such difficulties are clearly likely to affect the child's relationship with peers but may also contribute to him being seen as disobedient. Thus, most 14-year-olds know that when a teacher says 'Would you like to come and see me after class', a choice is not really being given. This may not be the case for some brain-injured children.

Memory impairments

Memory impairment, following BI, can be a source of strain for others in the family (Rivara *et al*, 1992) and is also likely to hamper academic progress, which is an important aspect of self-esteem for many children (Berk 1991). In addition, children who lose track of conversations because of memory problems or forget important events in others' lives are hardly likely to endear themselves to peers.

Attentional problems

Attentional problems may affect the child's behaviour in a number of areas. Such problems may be linked to brain-injured children being easily distracted and having difficulty following through or finishing things, both of which can be a source of strain to many parents (Rivara *et al*, 1992). Attentional problems appear to be linked to high levels of activity and impulsivity, which cause problems for parents and affect peer relationships (Berk 1991). In addition, the ability to switch attention during conversations as well as filter out irrelevant distractions is important if discussions are to proceed smoothly. Furthermore, attentional problems are likely to hamper academic progress and so affect self-esteem.

Perceptual and reasoning difficulties

The importance of perceptual difficulties for psychosocial functioning lies in the effect such deficits may have on physical abilities (such as eye and hand coordination) and academic progress which, as noted previously, are important for self-esteem. Deficits in reasoning abilities would be expected to affect children's academic progress and, therefore, their self-esteem.

Processing of socio-emotional information

Research with adults indicates that BI can affect the ability to accurately perceive and comprehend emotional information provided by others via lexical, facial, and prosodic channels (Borod 1992). Similarly, compared to controls, head-injured children tend to have greater difficulty in recognizing facial expressions and perform more poorly on a social perspective-taking task (Pettersen 1991). Such deficits are clearly likely to affect the ability of brain-injured children to relate to others and may also contribute to behaviour problems. For example, if it is not noticed that others are angered or disgusted by a particular behaviour then it may be more likely to be repeated.

Executive function deficits

Much complex human behaviour, especially social behaviour, appears to require executive function (Pennington and Ozonoff 1996). The definition of executive function is, however, underspecified and provisional but can, briefly, be defined as 'the ability to maintain an appropriate problem-solving set for the attainment of a future goal' (Pennington and Ozonoff 1996). Specifically, such goal-directed activity requires selective and sustained attention to salient stimuli, the recognition and selection of potential goals, the formulation and implementation of a reasonable plan to obtain the chosen goal, monitoring progress towards the chosen goal via the utilization of feedback, and inhibition of inappropriate responses (Mateer and Williams 1991). The concept of executive functioning, therefore, is closely related to the idea of a limited-capacity central processing system; has clear links with the domains of attention, reasoning, and problem-solving; and a central aspect of the concept is that of context-specific action selection, particularly if strongly competing, but context-inappropriate responses, are possible (Pennington and Ozonoff 1996). Deficits of executive functioning are linked to a number of problems, including disinhibition (including being stimulus-bound or captured by – possibly irrelevant – environmental, internal, or action-generated stimuli), perseveration (i.e. continuing in a course of action that is no longer appropriate), failure to initiate appropriate activity, failure to maintain effort and attention over time, failure to recognize or utilize feedback, and failure to independently modulate activity (Mateer and Williams 1991). Such deficits would be expected to impair performance in social situations and contribute to emotional and behavioural difficulties. For instance, children may swear at each other in the playground but not at teachers or parents. In these contexts such a response is inappropriate and will usually be inhibited, but may not be following BI.

Executive dysfunction is thought to be largely due to damage to the frontal lobes, the part of the brain which is thought to be particularly susceptible to damage, following a closed HI. Although damage to different parts of the frontal lobe may result in different behavioural syndromes in adults, a review of various published case studies of nine children who had sustained definite damage to the frontal lobes (Pennington and Bennetto 1993) noted a common pattern of severe conduct problems following such damage. Seven of the children demonstrated at least one of the following: physical violence towards others, illegal behaviour (e.g. theft), and significant difficulties in forming and maintaining meaningful interpersonal relationships. It is clearly important, therefore, that when a child suffers a BI, executive functions are formally assessed, otherwise there is a danger of the child simply being labelled 'bad'. A number of adults with documented frontal lesions have, however, performed quite well on putative tests of executive function but also shown difficulties in everyday life, indicative of executive dysfunction (Pennington and Ozonoff 1996). The individual's performance in natural, unstructured settings also, therefore, needs to be assessed.

Psychological reaction

The BI survivor may have a psychological reaction to the accident *per se* and any cognitive or other losses he has suffered because of the injury, and also needs to learn to cope with others' reactions to any acquired disabilities.

Psychological reaction to the accident

It has been suggested that following traumatic brain injury (TBI), post-traumatic stress disorder (PTSD) may develop in both children and adults. The diagnostic criteria for PTSD for adults are as follows:

- first, experience of a traumatic event outside the range of normal human experience.
- second, that the traumatic event be re-experienced, for example, via recurrent and intrusive recollections, dreams, or symbolically.
- third, persistent avoidance of stimuli associated with the precipitating event or emotional numbing.
- fourth, persistent symptoms of increased arousal not present before the trauma, such as problems falling or remaining asleep or hypervigilance.

Children appear to exhibit a similar pattern of symptoms following exposure to a severe stressor, although emotional numbing may not occur (Yule 1994).

Many TBI survivors, however, appear to have no conscious recollection of events around the time of the accident, amnesia which is believed to be organically mediated, and the diagnosis of PTSD, requires that the traumatic event is re-experienced. Such TBI survivors should, therefore, be protected against the development of PTSD and there is some empirical support for this hypothesis (Sbordone and Liter 1995). It has, however, been argued that whilst there may be no declarative memory of the accident, there may be an implicit memory of it which influences future behaviour (Layton and Wardi-Zonna 1995). For instance, one patient who was in a coma for 4 days following an accident for which she said she had no conscious recollection, described being haunted by images of motorcycles colliding and had other PTSD symptoms. Whilst, therefore, PTSD may be less likely to occur where there is no conscious memory of the accident, it may still do so. In addition, children with mild HI who can remember the accident may develop PTSD. In this light, it is important to note that children may be very reluctant to talk about traumatic events (Yule 1994) which may, mistakenly, be taken to indicate they cannot remember the event.

Whether or not there is any memory of the accident (implicit or declarative), it seems unreasonable to expect that having an accident which could have resulted in death will not have any emotional impact on the individual. Certainly, some children who have been seen clinically after a severe BI, who have no conscious recollection of the accident have been preoccupied with death. For example, one adolescent began drawing gravestones with his name on, much to his parents' distress. Symptoms such as a sense of foreshortened future, hypervigilance, and nightmares are, therefore, understandable. Although it is not shown in Fig. 9.1, should PTSD occur following BI it would be expected to affect performance on tests of concentration/ attention and memory.

Psychological reaction to losses

Little research has been done into how BI survivors (adults or children) cope with any losses they suffer because of the injury. It has, however, been noted that adult survivors tend to become depressed as more realistic self-awareness develops, which can be seen as grieving for the losses incurred, and thus, a normal part of an adjustment process (Ponsford 1995). As will be discussed later, however, there may, particularly in children, be a lack of awareness of some losses (such as loss of attentional abilities), following BI, which is likely to complicate any mourning or grieving process.

Children are, nevertheless, usually aware of changes such as having to attend a different school, being no longer able to keep up with other children academically, and having lost friends. Awareness of such losses may trigger a variety of feelings. Thus, a child may become frustrated and angry when he has difficulty performing a skill that he had mastered prior to the injury. A child who is aware that others are often angry at him (although without necessarily knowing why) may become anxious in social situations. A child who can no longer get a place in a sports team may become depressed. As with the parents of brain-injured children (see Chapter 11), loss reactions may be episodic and triggered by reminders of what was or could have been. For instance, one adolescent had such a reaction when he found some school reports that predated his injury. From these reports, his considerable loss of academic ability was very clear. He also had a loss reaction when his old friends went to university. He was aware that, but for the injury, he would have done likewise. Loss reactions can, therefore occur long after the injury has been sustained.

Self-esteem

As discussed previously, the low self-esteem found in children with BI is likely to be largely due to the effect of acquired difficulties on academic and physical abilities, coupled with a loss of friendships. In addition, being told off frequently for inappropriate behaviour is likely to affect self-esteem. There are, however, developmental changes in self-perception (Berk 1991) which also need to be taken into account. Thus, the self-judgements of 4 year-olds tend to be inordinately high and do not reflect objective evidence or others' opinions of them. Brain injury suffered at this age may not, therefore, have a large and immediate impact on self-esteem. The deficits acquired, however, may affect the child's subsequent academic progress and the development of social and physical abilities. Only as the child develops and becomes more aware of his abilities in relation to objective evidence and other children, may self-esteem be affected. Similarly, a child who suffers a BI at the age of 10 years, may immediately be aware of a loss of academic and sporting abilities. Not until adolescence, however, may he become aware of the implications of the injury for being able to get dates, and suffer a loss of self-esteem in this particular domain.

It is important to note that there may be a cumulative effect over time of cognitive and other impairments on academic progress. Following BI, a child may, therefore, increasingly fall behind his peers academically with a consequent steady, rather than precipitous, decline in self-esteem. The limited research which has been done in this area (Andrews *et al.* 1993) suggests that, following a moderate or severe HI, there is a significant loss of self-esteem in a number of domains. This includes self-esteem linked to the child's relationship with his parents. This possibly reflects children's aware-ness of the problems that they cause their parents.

Stigmatization

As well as having to deal with the loss of abilities and deficits, the BI survivor also has to learn to cope with society's response to disability (Pollack 1994).

Attitudes towards people with a disability appear to include the attribution of negative characteristics (e.g. stupidity) towards them, a rejection of intimacy with them, and an unwillingness to interact with them – attitudes which appear to be quite well established by the age of 8 years. In particular, few people report being willing to marry a person with a disability. The precise nature of the prejudice the brain-injured individual faces may depend upon the particular disability; for instance, physical disabilities may elicit name-calling. Many of the disabilities that BI causes, however, such as memory problems, are not immediately obvious to others but may only be detectable via repeated interaction. This may be a source of confusion and frustration to others, who may label the BI survivor as being lazy or uncaring. It is of course possible for BI survivors to explain to others the cause of the problem. However, brain injury is a condition which appears, *per se*, to be a source of stigmatization (Pollack 1994). People may not know what to expect of the brain injured individual and, therefore, become anxious and so avoid social contact with him. Certainly some brain-injured children have been told by peers 'My mum/dad says I shouldn't play with you because you're brain damaged'.

Psychological reaction to minor HI

As noted previously, there is some controversy concerning the likelihood of a minor HI causing emotional and behavioural problems. Obviously, such an injury does not usually produce cognitive or other deficits that could result in major loss reactions; indeed, cognitive impairments are usually mild and transient. The individual may, however, be immediately aware of such impairments. It has been found that, in adults, high levels of emotional changes can follow such injuries and, in particular, obsessive/compulsive symptoms may develop, which may be due to an awareness of cognitive inefficiencies and the need to develop compensatory techniques (see Morton and Wehman 1995). Thus, being aware of a newly acquired tendency to forget things may lead to anxiety and compulsive checking. Mild BI may also receive less environmental acceptance with the survivor being told to 'pull his socks up' or accused of malingering. Whether or not such effects occur with children, however, remains to be determined.

Brain injury

Although depression following BI in adults may result from the losses the survivor has suffered, it may also be due to injury to the parts of the brain involved in the experience of mood, particularly in the early stages following the injury, whilst there is also evidence that anxiety seen following BI to adults, may be due to damage to the neural structures regulating this emotion (see Miller 1991). There is, however, some controversy concerning the use of pharmacotherapy with brain-injured adults (Ponsford 1995) and this controversy is likely to be greater concerning the use of such therapy with children, particularly if the drugs which are likely to be prescribed may be associated with potentially significant side-effects.

Difficulties in social interaction

Evidence that children do have difficulties in social interaction, following BI, comes largely from parental reports. In one study (Pettersen 1991), children with HI were reported to have difficulty with the following:

- responding verbally and positively to the good fortune of others
- responding to hints or direct cues in the conversation
- monopolizing and interrupting conversations
- ending conversations appropriately
- apologizing for hurting others' feelings
- understanding the point of others' jokes or humorous remarks.

Another study (Papero *et al*, 1993) noted that head-injured children had difficulty in remembering to say please without prompting, keeping secrets, and in not asking embarrassing questions. These failings are likely to stem from cognitive deficits such as difficulties with attention, memory, abstract reasoning, and, in particular, executive functions. Emotional and behavioural problems such as hyperactivity, anxiety and depression are also, however, likely to impair social interaction.

Social rejection of, and social withdrawal by, the child with brain injury

It seems clear that some children with BI show behavioural and cognitive difficulties which are associated with peer rejection in the general population. Thus, children who show high rates of conflict, aggression, hyperactive–distractible behaviour, and immature forms of play along with deficits in social-cognitive skills, such as poor perspective-taking abilities and difficulty generating prosocial solutions to hypothetical social problems, are often rejected by peers. Similarly, sadness, difficulty coping with teasing, and a lack of a sense of humour are associated with low social status (Berk 1991). Some brain-injured children appear to notice that they are having difficulties in social interaction or are being rejected (although without necessarily knowing why) and so withdraw socially. Some children also appear to find it difficult to cope with the loss of social status that their difficulties may cause and so withdraw from activities.

Social isolation

That adults tend to become socially isolated, following BI, is well-established (Morton and Wehman 1995). In the one study (Andrews *et al*. 1993) that has been done with children following HI, significantly higher levels of self-reported loneliness were found in moderately and severely injured children compared to controls. Once social isolation is established it appears to be quite stable, and when children have given a peer a label, such as being hostile, the label tends to stick and blaming quickly occurs (Berk 1991).

Clinical experience suggests that if brain-injured children do lose old friends they may well gravitate towards other rejected children. These new friends can take advantage of their deficits by, for example, encouraging them to engage in antisocial acts.

If the BI is sufficiently severe then the child may have to change school. Not only does this mean the potential loss of old friends but also the need to learn to relate to new schoolmates. Attempting to join a well-established social group can be a daunting task in itself, but also occurs at a time when the skills needed to do so have probably been impaired.

DENIAL

Denial of deficits/disabilities appears to be common following BI in adults, two forms of which have been identified, these being neurogenic and psychogenic (Pollack 1994). Neurogenic denial has an organic basis and results from damage to areas of the brain governing subjective awareness and appreciation of performance, ambition, and concern. Psychogenic denial, on the other hand, has been referred to as motivated unawareness and is thought to reflect a psychological defence mechanism that functions to reduce the anxiety that would be experienced if the deficits and disabilities which threaten the sense of self were acknowledged. Not only may current disabilities/deficits and likely future limitations be denied but past abilities may be minimized, thus reducing the loss suffered (Deaton 1986). Some problems, such as motor impairment, may be acknowledged more readily than others, such as cognitive, behavioural, and emotional problems. This may be because these latter problems are less objectifiable and less easily separated from one's sense of self. It may also, however, be due to such problems requiring more capacity for self-reflection. Distinguishing between these two forms of denial clinically may not be easy but may be done by analysing the survivor's reaction to being shown (progressively, respectfully, and cautiously) his limitations (Prigatano 1994). If denial is organically mediated, survivors may be surprised by their deficits whereas in psychogenic denial, resistance may be shown to the process.

It seems likely that the picture will be more complex for children than for adults because of developmental limitations in self-awareness. The use of psychogenic denial suggests that the individual has a reasonably accurate and sophisticated appreciation of his pre-morbid personality and abilities and there is some awareness of how these have changed following BI. Children's self-awareness, particularly of their personality, may, however, be relatively unsophisticated and inaccurate, at least until the age of 11 years (Berk 1991). Children's lack of awareness of some changes, following BI, may well, therefore, reflect developmental limitations rather than denial. The little available research into children's awareness *per se* of deficits, following HI, suggest a considerable degree of ignorance and a tendency to concentrate on motor impairments (Jacobs 1993). Nevertheless, there were also indicators in this study of the use of psychogenic denial by the children.

Whatever the origin of the denial, it can have both beneficial and detrimental effects. Some potential beneficial effects of denial are shown in Fig. 9.1. Brain-injured individuals may, for example, deny that they have suffered a loss of social status and so a tendency to withdraw socially may not occur, reducing the likelihood of their becoming socially isolated. In addition, if losses of ability are denied then feelings of anxiety and depression and loss of self-esteem may be avoided. Such denial may, however, also prevent the BI survivor engaging in rehabilitation, thus leading to less recovery of skills. The consequences of denial therefore need to be considered before intervening (Deaton 1986). For example, some survivors may verbally deny deficits while continuing to engage in activities aimed at recovering lost skills, in which case, challenging the denial may be unnecessary and, indeed, inappropriate. Furthermore, denial of likely future limitations may result in increased hope and the survivor working harder, and perhaps achieving, goals that initially seem unrealistic.

TREATMENT

Interventions to help the child with emotional, behavioural, and social problems following a BI are obviously going to be based on an assessment of potential cause(s), such as those outlined in Fig. 9.1. Disentangling the possible reasons for the problems, however, may prove difficult and sometimes be impossible. For example, a child may present as being depressed and may well have reason for being so, given the losses he has suffered. The depression may, at least partly, however, have an organic basis. In many cases the aetiology is likely to be multifactorial and so require multiple interventions. Thus, a disinhibited child may be seen individually for anger management training whilst the parents carry out a behavioural programme aimed at reducing temper outbursts.

Potential interventions with children and their families are discussed below. It should, however, be borne in mind that research into the effectiveness of the techniques described with, specifically, brain-injured children, is very limited.

Interventions with children

There are a number of possible ways to intervene individually with children, following a BI. Some of the major approaches are detailed below.

Education

It is increasingly recognized that open and honest communication with children who have medical conditions is essential to promote their psychological well-being. There appears to have been only one small-scale, classroom based study of children's knowledge of their BI, and this found such knowledge to be poor (Jacobs 1993). Thus, children were often ignorant of how their injury was caused and how long they had been in a coma. Other confusions, e.g. between a 'shunt' (an abbreviated term for a ventriculoperitoneal shunt, often used to treat hydrocephalus) and a 'trache' (an abbreviated term for a tracheostomy, often used to help breathing, particularly if the child had been on the intensive care unit), were also noted. In addition, the children's knowledge of normal brain function was found to be very limited and some did not seem to know that failure to remember how the injury was sustained was normal. Although the children did appear to be aware of their physical disabilities, and some knew it was harder for them to learn since the injury, awareness of cognitive problems was very poor. The children were, therefore, provided with accurate information about how the injury was caused and the duration of their coma so they could develop personal narratives about their lives. They were also given factual information about the role of the brain and their disabilities were discussed with them.

In teaching the child about BI, his level of understanding obviously needs to be taken into account. A book about BI has been produced for children (see Chapter 11) which may be helpful in this respect. Nevertheless, some concepts are likely to be beyond some children. For older children, metaphors or images that make concepts meaningful may be useful (Ylvisaker and Szekeres 1987). Thus, a sports-minded young adolescent may find the metaphor that the frontal lobes act as a sort of sports coach makes executive dysfunction more understandable. It is important that informed consent is obtained from parents since some misconceptions children may hold, for example that a BI can heal in the same way a broken bone may mend, may be challenged in therapy. Similarly, education is likely to make children more aware of their deficits. In the short term this may be distressing to the child. If, however, children do not understand their difficulties then a vicious cycle may develop in which socially inappropriate behaviour results in negative feedback, but there is no understanding of why or how to correct such behaviours.

Individual psychotherapy

With adults, individual psychotherapy following BI may have a number of aims, including helping survivors cope with the losses (cognitive, motor, social, occupational/educational, etc.) they have suffered because of the BI and acquire a new sense of self; the resolution of pre-morbid psychological problems which can no longer be coped with because of reduced abilities and capacities (Miller 1991); and the exploration of phenomenological issues raised by the BI such as 'Why did this happen to me?', 'Will I be normal again?', and 'Is life worth living after brain injury?' (Prigatano 1994, p.175). The value of at least some forms of individual psychotherapy to brain-injured individuals has, however, been questioned since insight-orientated therapy (such as psychodynamic therapy) requires attributes, such as the ability to tolerate frustration and anxiety, that may be impaired by BI (see Pollack 1994). In particular, there has been concern (Miller 1991) that insight-orientated psychotherapy would precipitate a catastrophic reaction in the survivor, resulting in him being overwhelmed by feelings. Whilst some survivors neuropsychological deficits may indeed suggest that insight-or-ientated psychotherapy is counter-indicated, it has been argued that psychotherapy has a vital role to play in rehabilitation following BI for most survivors' (Prigatano 1994). Furthermore, it may be possible to modify even insight-orientated therapies to better fit the abilities and capacities of the BI survivor. Such modifications might include briefer sessions (because of attentional problems), more frequent sessions (because of memory problems), interpretations being postponed or given tentatively (because of difficulty tolerating anxiety), interpretations being immediately followed by cognitive restructuring (because of cognitive disorganization), and the avoidance of open-ended anxiety provoking comments and questions (Miller 1991; Pollack 1994). In general, it is likely to be more difficult to establish a therapeutic alliance, and therapy is likely to be more concrete and directive and involve more educational components (particularly in the early stages) than would be usual and so proceed more slowly.

There has been much less research (and debate in the literature) into the use of individual psychotherapy with children and adolescents, following BI. Indeed, there would only appear to be one published case study of psycho-dynamic therapy with a brain-injured child (Judd 1988). It can, however, play an important part in rehabilitation for many children although, as with adults, it may need to be modified to take account of the survivor's abilities.

The concerns of brain-injured children and adolescents that can emerge during therapy may be similar to those of adults but need also to be seen in the light of developmental issues. For example, adult BI survivors may feel that they have been punished for something they have done wrong, even following unavoidable accidents (Pollack 1994). Such thinking appears to come more readily to children, particularly under the age of 7 years. Other issues may be less likely to occur with children. For example, younger children may be less prone to wondering if life is worth living after suffering a BI, although clinical experience suggests this can occur in adolescents, which can be extremely upsetting for parents. The particular significance of an impairment may also change with development. Thus, younger children may be concerned that a motor impairment sets them apart from their peers and restricts their physical activities. In adolescence, their main concern may be that the impairment makes them less attractive to potential sexual partners.

Post-traumatic stress disorder

Children need to know that PTSD is a normal reaction to an abnormal event and be provided with a safe, supportive environment in which to discuss and/or write and draw about the traumatic event. Therapeutic sessions which are too brief may sensitize rather than desensitize children to the trauma. Children can also be taught relaxation techniques and to identify stimuli which trigger anxiety. Sleeping problems should be tackled early on since sleep deprivation is likely to impair the child's ability to function in everyday situations and so compound problems. If the child has difficulty getting to sleep then the use of relaxing routines before going to bed may help. Music may help mask or distract the child from intrusive thoughts which prevent sleep onset. Nightmares linked to accidents can be treated via relaxation and systematic desensitization coupled with teaching positive self-statements and story-line alteration, i.e. the nightmare is recounted with a different, happy ending (Yule 1994).

Anger management

A cognitive-behaviourial approach for anger control for adults with BI has been outlined (see Ponsford 1995) in which detailed records are kept to identify triggers and patterns of anger outbursts and alternative, appropriate strategies are developed to handle such situations. The acronym 'ANGER' is used to summarize the approach, which involves the individual learning to:

• Anticipate trigger situations (who, where, and when)

- Notice signs of anger increasing (physical and affective)
- Go through a temper routine (consciously use relaxation techniques and breathing exercises and think of alternative strategies to deal with the situation)
- Extract himself from the situation (if all else fails)
- Record the outcome (to learn from the experience).

Appropriate social and assertiveness skills are also taught to the BI survivor. Where, however, there is little external impetus for change, or the survivor has poor self-monitoring skills, or the problem is long-standing, such a strategy may not be effective. Similar cognitive-behavioural techniques have been used with children without BI who have anger problems, but may only be suitable for children above the age of about 10 years (Spence 1995). This age limit may be higher in the case of children with BI, owing to their likely reduced cognitive abilities.

Social skills training

A comprehensive package to teach children social skills has recently been developed (Spence 1995). Included in the package are questionnaires on the child's social skills and competence (to be completed by the child, parent, and teacher), a brief test to assess the child's ability to perceive facial expressions and gestures, and a chart – useful in helping identify social difficulties during observation of the child. Interventions outlined in the package are aimed at teaching children micro-level social skills (such as appropriate eye contact) and macro-level skills (such as starting conversations) along with social-cognitive skills. These latter skills encompass social perception (such as attending to relevant social cues and social perspective-taking skills), social problem-solving skills (identifying the nature of the problem, determining goals, generating possible responses, etc.), and self-monitoring skills (such as accurately labelling one's own behaviour).

The package may be helpful in identifying the nature of any social difficulties shown by brain-injured children and provide interventions to help alleviate these difficulties. The social perception and social problem-solving aspects would appear to be particularly relevant. It has, however, proved difficult to teach children social perception skills, and, in addition, social skills taught in one setting may not generalize to other settings (Spence, 1995). Given evidence in brain-injured children of poor social perception skills and a tendency for skills taught in one setting not to generalize to other settings, particular emphasis may need to be placed on these aspects when using the package with such children.

Interventions with parents

The main thrust of treatment interventions is likely to be aimed at parents because it is they who have to deal with the child on a daily basis. Indeed in some cases, unfortunately, they may have to care for the child for the rest of their lives. In addition, some interventions with the child are unlikely to be successful without parental support. Thus, teaching a child anger-management skills is unlikely to be effective if temper outbursts continue to be rewarded at home.

Education

Educating parents about BI and related issues is very important. General topics which should be covered in any educational programme for parents are outlined in Chapter 11. Parents, and other family members also, however, need to be educated about the specific neuropsychological deficits shown by the brain-injured child. This particularly applies to executive dysfunction, which many parents appear to find confusing. In addition, because of the structured environment that is usually provided for young children by their parents, the consequences of such deficits may be minimal in this age group. As a result, parents may see little reason to intervene to improve executive functions. However, in view of evidence that executive dysfunction appears to be linked to poor outcome, it is possible that early intervention may prevent future problems developing. Possible strategies for improving executive functions have been described elsewhere (Ylvisaker and Szekeres 1989). Furthermore, the way in which brain-injured children are managed generally by parents may need to be altered to take into account the child's deficits by, for example, providing more structure and routine.

Behaviour management

Behaviour management is likely to be the main approach taken with children with BI and is described in detail elsewhere (Deaton 1994). Such an approach often needs to be implemented before other treatment strategies are tried since children with severe behaviour problems are likely to drain the parents' resources and result in a deterioration in the relationship between the child and parents (Leichtman 1992). The following stages in the implementation of a behavioural programme have been described (Deaton 1994).

First, the problem (or target) behaviour must be defined. The people involved in implementing the programme need to agree on a precise, detailed description of the behaviour to be changed. There should be agreement between the people implementing the programme (such as family members, teachers, and all rehabilitation staff) that the behaviour is a problem and should be tackled. The BI survivor should be involved at this and other stages and agree that the behaviour needs to change.

Second, a baseline assessment needs to be carried out to identify the function, cause, and rate of the target behaviour along with other salient characteristics such as intensity and duration. During this stage, information is gained on the events preceding (antecedents) and following (consequences) the target behaviour which indicate why the behaviour occurs. Antecedents can include cognitions, emotions, settings, or behaviours. Consequences can be viewed as being positive (which serve to reinforce the behaviour and make it more likely it will occur in the future) or negative (and so decrease the likelihood of future occurrence). It is, however, the child's perception of the consequences which is most important. Thus, the brain-injured child may be desperate to make friends and believe that certain behaviours cause his peers enjoyment and increase his popularity. To the outside observer, however, it may be clear that he is being used by peers as a source of amusement. A behaviour may also be found to serve a number of different functions. Thus, a child may hit peers to both obtain desired toys and stop them teasing him. In addition, once a behaviour is established, reinforcement may only need to be intermittent in order for it to be maintained. Baseline assessment may therefore need to be prolonged in order to identify factors that serve to maintain the behaviour. This can be a source of frustration to parents; however, premature intervention is likely to lead to failure. During baseline assessment it may also become clear that the behaviour is not as great a problem as was initially thought as there is a tendency to see intense behaviours (such as temper tantrums) as being more frequent than is actually the case.

In the third stage the resources available for behavioral intervention need to be identified. Resources may include the assets of the brain-injured survivor, such as memory, motivation, and learning ability. Assessment of the family's assets such as knowledge of BI, the time and energy available from family members, and their ability to be consistent in implementing any behavioural programme is likely to be very important. Programmes can take a considerable time to be effective and, particularly with BI survivors, need to be very consistently applied – by all those involved in caring for the child. As discussed previously, parents can have strong feelings of guilt and sympathy for the child, which may interfere with their ability to carry out a behavioural programme. Such feelings therefore need to be addressed before it is implemented. A programme which is begun but not carried through is likely to result in feelings of frustration, helplessness, and even failure on the part of the parents, and to confuse the child, possibly resulting in a deterioration in his behaviour.

Fourth, potential strategies for changing the child's behaviour need to be identified. Thus, a child who refuses to comply with requests may be given written instructions, rewarded for completing tasks, given time out (from positive reinforcement) for not following the request, removed to a less stressful situation, or suffer a loss of privileges, etc. There is often a tendency to concentrate on simply decreasing undesirable behaviour, such as hitting peers, and prosocial alternatives to such behaviour need to be developed and rewarded. Rewards are likely to be highly individual to the child, may change with time, and need to be given immediately after the desired behaviour for maximum effectiveness.

Fifth, the chosen strategy must be implemented and evaluated via ongoing collection of data. Parents need to be forewarned that in some cases the problem behaviour is likely to escalate before it diminishes. For instance, if temper tantrums have been effective for the child in the past, these are likely to become more prolonged and intense at the start of the programme. If parents acquiesce to these tantrums all the child will have learned is that he should escalate his behaviour in order to achieve what he wants. Concrete feedback in the form of graphs or charts may be needed for the child with memory problems. Continual evaluation will help determine if the intervention is being successful and, if not, help identify possible reasons for its failure such as inconsistent implementation.

The final stages involves the maintenance and generalization of desirable behaviours. This demands a gradual shift in control of the behaviour back to the child and away from external sources, and a fading of reinforcement. Rewards need to become less concrete, less frequently given, and less artificial, but such changes need to be very gradual. Behaviours taught in one setting to a child with BI may be less likely to generalize to other settings. Skills may therefore need to be taught in a variety of settings.

Once parents and others have learned behaviour management techniques, they can be applied to a variety of problems and so reduce the need for professional consultation. The time and effort needed by parents to learn to use such techniques should not, however, be underestimated.

Family counselling/therapy

It is likely that when a child suffers a BI the whole family is affected. Premorbid difficulties in family relationships may also contribute to any behavioural problems the child had prior to the injury and affect his post-injury adjustment. For these reasons, work with the family as a whole may be necessary if the brain-injured child's behaviour problems are to be successfully tackled. These issues are discussed further in Chapter 11.

REFERENCES

Andrews, T. K., Johnson, D. A., and Rose, F. D. (1993). *Social and behavioural problems following closed head injury in children*. Paper presented at the BPS meeting *Neuropsychological aspects of brain injury and recovery*. St. Andrews University, Scotland, September 1993.

Asarnow, R. F., Satz, P., Light, R., Lewis, R., and Neumann, E. (1991). Behaviour problems and adaptive functioning in children with mild and severe closed head injury. *Journal of Pediatric Psychology*, **16**, 543–55.

Berk, L. E. (1991). *Child Development (2nd edn)*. Allyn and Bacon, Needham Heights, MA.

Borod, J. C. (1992). Interhemispheric and intrahemispheric control of emotion: a focus on unilateral brain damage. *Journal of Consulting and Clinical Psychology*, **60**, 339–48.

Brown, G., Chadwick, O., Shaffer, D., Rutter, M., and Traub, M. (1981). A prospective study of children with head injuries. III. Psychiatric sequelae. *Psychological Medicine*, **11**, 63–8

Deaton, A. V. (1986). Denial in the aftermath of traumatic head injury: its manifestations, measurement and treatment. *Rehabilitation Psychology*, **31**, 231–40.

Deaton, A. V. (1994). Changing the behaviors of students with acquired brain injury. In *Educational dimensions of acquired brain injury* (ed, R. C. Savage and G. F. Wolcott). PRO-FD, Inc., Austin, TX.

Deaton, A. V. and Waaland, P. (1994). Psychosocial effects of acquired brain injury. In *Educational dimensions of acquired brain injury* (ed. R. C. Savage and G. F. Wolcott). PRO-FD, Inc., Austin, TX.

Dennis, M. (1991). Frontal-lobe function in childhood and adolescence: a heuristic for assessing attention regulation, executive control, and the intentional states important for social discourse. *Developmental Neuropsychology*, **7**, 327–58.

Donders, J. (1992). Pre-morbid behavioural and psychosocial adjustment in children with traumatic brain injury. *Journal of Abnormal Child Psychology*, **20**, 233–46.

Jacobs, M. P. (1993). Limited understanding of deficit in children with brain dysfunction. *Neuropsychological Rehabilitation*, **3**, 341–66.

Judd, D. (1988). The hollow laugh: An account of the first six months in therapy with a brain-damaged boy. *Journal of Child Psychotherapy*, **14**, 79–92.

Layton, B. S. and Wardi-Zonna, K. (1995). Post-traumatic stress disorder with neurogenic amnesia for the traumatic event. *The Clinical Neuropsychologist*, **9**, 2–10.

Lehr, E. (1990). *Psychological management of traumatic brain injuries in children and adolescents*, p.160 Aspen Publishers Inc., Rockville, MD.

Leichtman, M. (1992). Psychotherapeutic interventions with brain-injured children and their families. I. Diagnosis and treatment planning. *Bulletin of the Menninger Clinic*, **56**, 321–37.

Mateer, C. A. and Williams, D. (1991). Effects of frontal-lobe injury in childhood. *Developmental Neuropsychology*, **7**, 359–76.

Miller, L. (1991). Psychotherapy of the brain-injured patient: principles and practices. *Cognitive Rehabilitation*, **9**, 24–30.

Morton, M. V. and Wehman, P. (1995). Psychosocial and emotional sequelae of individuals with traumatic brain injury: a literature review and recommendations. *Brain Injury*, **9**, 81–92.

Papero, P. H., Prigatano, G. P., Snyder, H. M., and Johnson, D. L. (1993). Children's adaptive behavioural competence after head injury. *Neuropsychological Rehabilitation*, **3**, 321–40.

Parker, G. (1990). The parental bonding instrument: a decade of research. *Social Psychiatry and Psychiatric Epidemiology*, **25**, 281–2.

Pelco, L., Sawyer, M., Duffield, G., Prior, M., *et al.* (1992). Premorbid emotional and behavioural adjustment in children with mild head injuries. *Brain Injury*, **6**, 29–37.

Pennington, B. F. and Bennetto, L. (1993). Main effects or transactions in the neuropsychology of conduct disorder? Commentary on 'the neuropsychology of conduct disorder'. *Development and Psychopathology*, **5**, 153–64.

Pennington, B. F. and Ozonoff, S. (1996). Executive functions and developmental psychopathology. *Journal of Child Psychology and Psychiatry*, **37**, 51–87.

Pettersen, L. (1991). Sensitivity to emotional cues and social behaviour in children and adolescents after head-injury. *Perceptual and Motor Skills*, **73**, 1139 –50.

Pollack, I.W. (1994). Individual psychotherapy. In *Neuropsychiatry of traumatic brain injury* (ed. J. M. Silver, S. C. Yudofsky, and R. F. Hales). American Psychiatric Press, Washington, DC.

Ponsford, J. (with Sloan, S. and Snow, P.) (1995). *Traumatic brain injury: rehabilitation for everyday adaptive living.* Laurence Erlbaum Associates Ltd. Hove.

Prigatano, G. P. (1994). Individuality, lesion location and psychotherapy after brain injury. In *Brain injury and neuropsychological rehabilitation* (ed. A-L. Christensen and B. P. Uzell) Laurence Erlbaum Associates, Hillsdale, N J.

Rivara, J. B. , Fay, G., Jaffe, K., Polissar, N., Shurtleff, H., and Martin, K. (1992). Predictors of family functioning one year following traumatic brain injury in children. *Archives of Physical Medicine and Rehabilitation*, **73**, 899–910.

Sbordone, R. J., and Liter, J. C. (1995). Mild traumatic brain injury does not produce post-traumatic stress disorder. *Brain Injury*, **9**, 405–12.

Spence, S. H. (1995). *Social skills training.* NFER-Nelson, Windsor.

Thomasgard, M. and Metz, W. P. (1993). Parental overprotection revisited. *Child Psychiatry and Human Development*, **24**, 67–80.

Ylvisaker, M. and Szekeres, S. F. (1989). Metacognitive and executive impairments in head-injured children and adults. *Topics in Language Disorders*, **9**, 34–49.

Yule, W. (1994). Post-traumatic stress disorder. In *Child and adolescent psychiatry: modern approaches* (ed. M. Rutter, E. Taylor, and L. Hersov) Blackwell Scientific Publications, Oxford.

10

Community liaison

Jackie Gregg, Richard Appleton, and Tony Baldwin

The aims of community liaison are to ensure that:

- early medical advice is submitted to the local education authority (LEA), if necessary, to ensure optimal educational provision
- the local community doctor and family doctor are regularly updated on the child's progress, so that local support is readily available for parents, siblings, and extended family
- the child's local community doctor, general practitioner, and therapists are briefed ready for the child's discharge.

In Liverpool, the head-injury rehabilitation team (HIRT) member responsible for community liaison is a consultant community paediatrician within the Trust. Her role is to look at the 'whole' child within the hospital *and* community settings.

Within our team, the community doctor chairs team meetings to address the child's social, emotional, health, and educational needs, as well as ensuring as smooth a transfer as possible from hospital to community care when the child is discharged home.

Community liaison will be considered during the three phases of a child's care:

- under the care of the team while an in-patient
- under the care of the team while an out-patient or day-patient
- discharge from the team.

The importance of community involvement stems from the statutory responsibilities of the community child health services.

COMMUNITY CHILD HEALTH SERVICES

Financial considerations and the new purchaser-provider split have resulted in clarification of the role of the community child health services. The BPA document *Community child health services: an information base for purchasers*

(BPA 1992) advises health authorities of the services that should be available, including services for preschool and schoolchildren, disadvantaged children, children with special needs, and also in the area of child protection. The report *Health needs of school age children'* (Polnay 1995) clarifies in detail the role of community doctors and nurses. The report advocates a named doctor for particular important aspects of community work, including work with children with special needs and 1993 Education Act advice.

It is recommended that every school has a named nurse and paediatrician with special training in the health of children and young people and in educational medicine. The Court report (1976) defined educational medicine as: 'The study and practice of child health and paediatrics in relation to the processes of learning. It requires an understanding of child development, the educational environment, the child's response to schooling, the disorders which interfere with the child's capacity to learn, and the special needs of the handicapped. Its practitioners need to work cooperatively with the teachers, psychologists and others who may be involved with the child and to understand the influences of family and social environment'.

The appointment of consultants in community child health has increased dramatically in the past 10 years, thereby fulfilling one of the recommendations of the Court report. The specially trained school nurse is an essential member of the school health team. The nurse works closely with the school doctor and teaching staff and spends a large proportion of the time in schools. She has an important role in health promotion, child protection, liaison with the primary health care team, and in providing nursing care for children with disabilities.

Emotional and behavioural problems are the largest cause of disability among children of school age. It is recognized that quite a significant proportion of a community paediatrician's work is involved with such problems, with the child and adolescent mental health services (where they exist) dealing with the most difficult cases.

Therapy services are an essential component in the assessment and management of children with special needs. Speech therapists, physiotherapists, and occupational therapists provide input for such children in the home, in clinics, and in special and mainstream schools. Their contribution to multidisciplinary teams is vital and close collaborative working with other health professionals is important. The creation of separate Trusts has tended to fragment the services for children unless there is one Trust encompassing all children's services. The British Paediatric Association (BPA) advocates a combined child health service (BPA 1991) in which hospital and community services are combined and managed together. Despite having considerable support, this has been achieved in only a few Trusts. Even a combined trust such as ours at Alder Hey is not ideal, as speech therapy services are not included. An additional anomaly is that health and social services both provide an occupational therapy service. Good management links are essential to ensure that occupational therapy services are therefore coordinated with no duplication.

The community doctor is in an ideal position to coordinate services for children, because of their background and training. Their statutory responsibilities mean that they are already doing this for many children in their area and have existing structures to make it work. The Education Acts of 1981 and 1993 require health authorities to notify the education authority of children likely to have special educational needs. This responsibility is passed on to the community child health services. A named doctor in each district is responsible to ensure that the Act is complied with and to coordinate information on the child's health needs to the LEA, as required. Local knowledge, child development teams, and close contact with colleagues in education and social services are already in place. Not infrequently, a large number of professionals may be involved with any one child. It is necessary that someone pulls it all together, to make sense of it for the family, and certainly to make sense of what is going on for the education department and social services.

UNDER THE CARE OF THE TEAM WHILE AN IN-PATIENT

Support for the family

A child admitted to hospital with a brain injury may initially be under the care of several specialists, including paediatric intensivists, neurosurgeons, and general surgeons. When the child's condition has stabilized and he is considered suitable for the team's involvement, the team is briefed on the background, the severity of the injury, and any social and family issues that are known. At this stage a summary letter, including all these details, is sent to the general practitioner and community paediatrician. It is essential for the primary health care team and community services to be kept fully informed so that they can provide adequate and, importantly, early support to the family.

In the initial stages, hospital staff usually provide most of the general support to children and their families. However, many parents frequently turn to their family doctor for clarification of certain issues related to the child's condition and care and also for support for themselves and their other children.

It is important that both hospital and community links are maintained. For example, a child involved as a passenger in a car accident might not have been the only family member injured. When a child is sick there is a tendency for parents to forget about their own health. Paediatric hospital staff may identify problems in parents and can help them obtain appropriate help through liaison with their family doctor.

Clearly, the flow of information is not all one way. The primary health care team and school health service themselves often have relevant information on the child and the family which can help to explain apparently unusual reactions by the family to the injury. Such insights can help hospital staff assist the parents to 'come to terms' with the injury. A complicated social background can at first be difficult to grasp but can explain unusual visiting patterns or behaviour of family members. Families frequently put on a brave face in hospital and give all the appearances of coping and understanding the situation, when in reality they are falling apart physically and emotionally. Professionals who have known the family for a long time can often detect this more readily than hospital staff. A quick telephone call to exchange information can go a long way to knowing how to deal with an upset parent.

The school doctor has an important role in informing the school of their pupil's condition, within the limits of confidentiality. The school may have been notified of the injury but have few details. They may simply have heard a report on the local radio or read something in the local paper which may be totally inaccurate. Rumours can quickly spread round a school, causing distress to both pupils and teachers. The facts are usually easier to deal with than rumour and uncertainty. Schoolfriends who wish to send cards may feel reticent until they have some definite information on the child's general condition.

The child's school may also feel partly responsible for the injury itself, as it is possible that their pupil sustained the head injury while in their care or while truanting from school. A classmate or friend who has been with the child when absent from school may be frightened of asking for help when trying to come to terms with their friend's injury. The school doctor is usually best placed, by working with teaching staff, to identify those in need of support and ensuring that they receive the appropriate services.

In the confusion and shock surrounding the acute injury and immediate period afterwards, siblings are, through necessity, often forgotten. Parents are by the sick child's bedside while brothers and sisters are expected to carry on attending school and behaving 'normally' while being looked after by friends or relatives. They too may have guilt feelings or just feel excluded as well as anxious and upset. They may turn to a trusted teacher to talk to. Teachers need to be aware of what is going on and how best to help the sibling cope with the situation. Ideally,they should be proactive and anticipate these problems, rather than being reactive and responding only when the problems or difficulties have developed. Other children can be very cruel and can say hurtful things about the injured child to their brother or sister, which a watchful teacher can curb or even prevent happening.

Notifying the local education authority

The community child health services have a statutory duty to notify the LEA of any child who may have special educational needs. As soon as it becomes apparent that the injured child will have residual difficulties and health problems which are likely to have an impact on their education, the team informs the local community paediatrician so that they can formally notify the LEA. Obviously, it may not be appropriate to initiate an educational assessment until the child's recovery has stabilized, as their needs will not have become apparent. However, the LEA may be able to proceed with some of the paperwork, including allocating an educational psychologist and perhaps identifying necessary resources. Although under the 1993 Education Act (Code of Practice) strict time limits have been put on each step of the assessment process, the statement of a child's special educational needs usually takes six months to complete. Health professionals and parents equally feel frustrated about this time scale. Most education authorities will provide emergency school placement and support before the statement has been prepared, but schools may not receive adequate resources until after the statement has been formally issued. It is felt that the earlier the education authority is notified about individual children, the better.

Preparing for discharge from hospital

Discharge from hospital is an important milestone in the recovery process, and good preparation is essential. For those with significant residual difficulties it is a traumatic event as the realities of those disabilities usually become more apparent in the outside world. Families can become very dependent on hospital staff and need to be given the confidence to realize that they will be able to cope with their child at home. Part of this includes explaining the rehabilitation process which will be carrying on for the child as an out-patient. It is important to know what will be expected of the child and also of the parents in that rehabilitation process. Some preparation and information on how the child is likely to react on discharge from hospital, and some strategies for handling their reactions should be provided for parents.

Information on this, as well as the programme of rehabilitation and the child's progress, are sent in a discharge summary to the different professionals within the community who are likely to be called upon to assist, advise, and treat the child, following discharge.

For some children, particularly those with significant residual difficulties, a planning meeting to prepare for discharge can be invaluable. This is particularly important for children who live some distance from the HIRT and are therefore unable to receive out-patient treatment from the team. For these children and their parents, the acute separation from hospital staff can be very traumatic. They need to feel that everything is in place, with named key people to whom they can turn for help, if and when necessary, when their child is referred back to the community.

The three key agencies who will be involved with a child on discharge from hospital are:

- community child health
- social services
- local education authority.

All have differing roles and responsibilities but there may be some overlap, and without careful planning, there may also be gaps in provision for families. A coordinated approach is therefore essential.

A planning meeting of all involved in the child's care, including parents, can identify what the child may need on discharge from hospital and ensure that these are provided. Adaptations to the home may be necessary and this is usually under the remit of social services. Unfortunately, this may take time to organize, but usually interim arrangements can be made, allowing the child to have short and, subsequently, increasingly long periods at home before final discharge. Assessment for such adaptations and aids are usually made by the social services' occupational therapist, following liaison with the occupational therapist member of the hospital team.

One particularly contentious issue, if the family needs assistance in the home, is whether this needs to be supplied by a trained nurse, a health-care assistant, or a care assistant. The sources of funding of these professionals are likely to be different and this may, therefore, have financial implications. For example, funding for a nurse and health care assistant may come from the health budget whereas the care assistant funding may come from the social-services budget. Hospital staff need to be aware of these distinctions in order to avoid giving inaccurate advice. It is understandable that parents who are expecting a trained nurse to help them look after their child may feel that a health-care assistant is totally unsuitable and have no confidence at all in that person. In fact, an appropriately trained and competent care assistant in particular aspects of the child's care may be much more able.

Schooling options are important; is the child going to return to his previous school, go to a special school, or a residential school? The family of a child with considerable needs who attends a day-school may need help after school hours, which could impact on the support that social services offer. Transport to and from school may also need to be considered as well as the skills of the person who may be needed to escort the child in the transport.

Factors to be considered:

- Does the child need extra help in addition to the resources already available in the school?

- Is an additional member of staff necessary?
- If the child has a particular health need, is a school nurse available?
- Do resources have to be allocated to provide a health-care assistant?

One specifically relevant example concerns health-care support for the child with a tracheostomy. Parents are trained in the care of a tracheostomy tube, and a trained health-care assistant is made available for any management that is necessary when the child is at school. If the child attends a special school there is likely to be such a health assistant on site. Obviously, they would have to be trained, as few people will have the necessary skills. However, funding would have to be found to train and employ a health assistant to support a child in mainstream school. If the child has a temporary tracheostomy which could be reversed at any time, it is not surprising that there could be some delay in arranging this. In addition, if the child attends a mainstream school, adaptations may be necessary. The parents will want to know how long that will take and the school will want to know who is going to pay for it – these are all very real issues when schools are now managing their own budgets.

It is obvious that a joint planning meeting between hospital and community health-care and educational staff can provide a very important exchange of information when planning for the child's discharge, particularly if he has significant residual difficulties. This involves a tremendous amount of work and preparation, including agreeing the sources of funding of different aspects of care and management. The ideal would be joint funding for a care package for children with disabilities, but this is not a reality at present in most districts. Families need to feel confident that all appropriate care is being made available for their child.

UNDER THE CARE OF THE TEAM WHILE AN OUT-PATIENT

On discharge from hospital, the rehabilitation process may continue on an out-patient or day-patient basis under the care and direction of the team; this will clearly depend on the severity of the brain injury. At this stage, a summary of the child's hospitalization and ongoing therapy and rehabilitation is sent to the primary care team and community services to update them on the child's progress and programme of out-patient rehabilitation.

The important areas for community liaison during this phase are:

- reviewing the child's progress
- resolving any problems that may subsequently arise following discharge
- updating the community and advising the education department regarding special educational needs

- passing information on to colleagues
- preparing the family for separation from the team

Review of progress

For children of school-age who live near enough to travel to the hospital on a daily basis, rehabilitation involves attending the hospital school and individual therapies, as appropriate. Many professionals can therefore be involved with any one child, so progress is discussed at weekly team meetings. This ensures that each member of the team is kept up to date with a child's overall progress and changes in his rehabilitation programme. The child is discussed more frequently between weekly team meetings, should problems arise and when he is ready for discharge.

The hospital school at Alder Hey is the largest in the country and provides teaching for 'long-stay' in-patients, either on the ward or in the school building (which is on the hospital site), and to out-patients who are receiving intensive therapies. Teaching staff have considerable expertise working with children with medical and surgical problems as well as experience in a wide range of learning difficulties and emotional disorders.

Attendance at the school gives the child the opportunity to continue their recovery in a protected environment, and also helps to build up their confidence in a classroom setting; it also functions as an assessment centre for a child's educational needs and abilities. Specific learning difficulties may be identified and delineated, with the information being passed on to the child's local education authority and a formal contribution being made to the educational assessment, if required.

The hospital school is under the control of Liverpool Education Authority, which facilitates transition to the most appropriate school placement for Liverpool children. Close links also exist between the hospital school and neighbouring education authorities. Educational psychologists from both local and other authorities are encouraged to visit the school and meet with teachers and children, if necessary.

Children are introduced to the hospital school prior to discharge so that they are familiar with staff and the layout of the school. Attendance is tailored to the child's educational needs and abilities as well as taking into account his overall medical status. Initially, a child may only be able to tolerate schooling for a few hours a day, and this usually starts while the child is still an in-patient. As soon as a child is able, he is encouraged to attend full-time. Children travelling from outside Liverpool may only attend for 2 or 3 days each week.

Flexibility is important, and teaching and therapies are planned to fit within the child's timetable of attendance. Therapists and the designated teacher for the team meet weekly to ensure that this timetable runs smoothly.

Medical and nursing input to the hospital school is provided by the local community services (which are a separate directorate within the hospital Trust). The school has a full-time health-care assistant on site. A school nursing sister is available to visit the school to give medication if required, and a senior nurse responsible for the special schools is available by bleep or telephone for emergencies or more specialist advice. Some children may have very particular and explicit nursing needs or require the care assistant to acquire additional skills. The health needs of each child is assessed prior to admission to the school to ensure that their needs can be met. Unfortunately this has not always been as straightforward as it sounds.

The hospital school has a named school doctor whose principal responsibility is in coordinating care for Liverpool residents. The doctor also has a wider remit in offering medical advice as necessary to the teachers and ensuring that the health needs of children in the school are being met.

Children recovering from brain injury often have numerous out-patient follow-up appointments with several different specialists. As the school is on the hospital site, attendance is much more convenient. Feedback is also easier; it is not unusual for teachers to raise concern about a particular aspect of the child's medical condition and the specialist facilities are readily available for assessment.

Transport to and from the school may be a problem for parents and, unfortunately, not all authorities are willing to provide or finance a taxi or hospital car. The LEA may argue (sometimes understandably) that the children are attending because of a medical need, and conversely, the health authority may argue (equally justifiably) that they are being educationally assessed in the school. Contact with the local community paediatrician is important as he or she is often best placed to resolve these issues.

Resolving problems

The rehabilitation process is a team effort, with the child and family at the core of the team. Children attending the hospital school have therapy within the school day and parents are always encouraged to attend but if they are unable to, the therapists try to keep them up to date by telephone or by letter. However, communication can sometimes be a problem and this can extend to failure to attend other out-patient clinics. This again emphasises the importance of the weekly team meetings to ensure a coordinated approach to the different therapies and teaching.

Behavioural problems in the child may only become apparent on discharge from hospital. Parents frequently feel powerless to discipline a child they have nearly lost. Team discussion on how best to advise the parents should ensure that appropriate – and importantly – consistent advice is given.

Guidance and support from the team's clinical and educational psychologists may be needed, including direct consultation with the family by the psychologist, if necessary. It is also important to brief the family doctor and community paediatrician, to whom the family may turn for advice. Behaviour problems may also, not infrequently, develop in a sibling, and the community doctor may be called upon to liaise between the school, the primary health care team, and the rehabilitation team to ensure that appropriate help is provided. It is often the schoolteacher who identifies such problems and is the first professional to alert the school doctor.

Not unexpectedly, progress does not always go according to plan, as recovery in a child is never entirely predictable. Close liaison with the many professionals involved can ensure speedy review of the child's progress and medical and surgical intervention as necessary.

An unanticipated difficulty and a problem which is likely to increase is the discharge from hospital of children colonized with methicillin-resistant *Staphylococcus aureus* (MRSA). MRSA is a strain of a bacterium that is commonly found in the nose of 30% of the population. To the normal healthy person, MRSA presents no problem at all. However, in a hospital setting the organism can gain access to sites of the body that it would normally not have access to, e.g. open wounds. Treatment is much more difficult as the organism is resistant to many of the commonly used antibiotics. It is safe to discharge patients who are colonized by the organism back into their families, provided they too are healthy. There is no bar to normal social contact such as returning to school. It is important to be clear on all these points as colonization can persist for many years (Duckworth 1990).

Unfortunately, recent documentary programmes on MRSA have produced alarm among the public, schools, and social services. Local written information should be made available for schools and social services, and a named person should be available by phone to answer queries and reassure the community, to ensure that there is no bar to the child being successfully reintegrated back into the community.

Updating the community and advising the education department

As soon as it is apparent that the child may have special educational needs, the senior community doctor and the LEA need to be notified. Under the 1993 Education Act, strict time-limits for the assessment process have been set. The community paediatrician must collate the health reports from all the medical and 'paramedic' personnel (including therapists) involved with the child and submit it to the LEA. It is important that these reports are submitted as rapidly as possible so as not to hold up or delay the educational assessment. The community doctor must be kept informed of all the different health professionals involved so that no important submissions of advice are omitted. The fully informed community doctor is more able to prepare the medical advice in a relevant and informative way for the LEA.

Passing information on to colleagues

When children are ready for discharge from the team a detailed summary is sent to the community paediatrician and general practitioner. Specific mention is made of any continuing problems (physical, behavioural, psychosocial, etc.) as well as outlining which therapies are still required. This is clearly important to ensure that the necessary appropriate provision can be made and the child's needs met.

Some children may need to continue with therapies once they are discharged from the team. In such cases, the team therapist will make contact with their community colleagues to discuss the work they have been doing with the child as well as sending detailed reports. Personal contact facilitates a much smoother hand-over and the community therapists are invited to meet the child and family in a joint therapy session prior to discharge.

Preparing the family for separation from the team

It will always be difficult for families to separate from professionals, particularly if they have been working with them for some months. Once a child and family become involved with the team, the function and role of the team is explained to ensure that the family will have no false expectations and understand that eventually they will be discharged to community follow-up. It is thus important for parents to see that good communication exists between the hospital and community and appropriate plans are drawn up for their child.

Separation may also be difficult for professionals (particularly the therapists) because of concern that the children will not receive adequate ongoing treatment due to a shortage of therapy services outside the hospital. This applies predominantly for paediatric occupational therapy and speech therapy. Some of the difficulties that the children may have can be specific and complicated; if the expertise to manage these difficulties is not available, this may limit the child's potential and optimal recovery from the injury.

DISCHARGE FROM THE TEAM

When the child is finally discharged from the team, future follow-up will be transferred to the local community services who will be responsible for ongoing coordination of care. By this stage the child should have been placed in the most appropriate community school. The community paediatrician is likely to be the person responsible for overseeing ongoing care and their role will include:

- follow-up and coordination of care
- ongoing advice to the LEA
- support for the family.

Follow-up and coordination of care

The outcome for children who have survived a brain injury covers the whole spectrum from complete recovery to severe disability. Children with a physical or sensory disability will have been identified early on while under the care of the hospital team. The children with more subtle problems may not become apparent until they are back at home or at school.

Children with a significant physical disability are likely to remain under review by a number of professionals both at the hospital and in the community. Specialists in the hospital such as the orthopaedic surgeon, paediatric neurologist, and orthotist may be dealing with only specific aspects of the child's problems. The child may also be receiving therapy from the community physiotherapist, occupational therapist, or speech therapist. The schoolchild may require input from a care assistant or school nurse. It is therefore important that the community paediatrician oversees the care of the whole child, and not just one or more specific problems. They must pull all the facets of the child's disability and care together to ensure that the child is receiving all appropriate services and nothing has been missed. It is clearly important for a single person to make sense of all this for the child and family. In addition the community paediatrician is able to assess and monitor the more general aspects of the child's well-being, including growth and nutrition. Delivery of this coordinated care will, in many districts, be centred round the child development centre (CDC) or child development team.

There is great variability from district to district in the availability of these facilities, the functioning of the CDC or team, and the individual professionals involved in the team (Bax and Whitmore 1991). It has been recommended that each district should have a CDC for the multidisciplinary assessment and therapy of children with disabilities. This has recently been endorsed in the report *Health needs of school age children* (Polnay 1995).

Follow-up of children with significant disabilities is likely to be shared between the community paediatrician and hospital-based paediatric neurologist, particularly if children have epilepsy or a neurological deficit, or both. Such shared care can be very advantageous to families by reducing the number of hospital visits and ensuring no gaps or deficiencies in the child's management; this obviously requires good communication between medical staff. They may also liaise closely with other hospital specialists, including audiology and ophthalmology and the relevant specialist teachers from the education department.

At Alder Hey, we maintain follow-up within the community for all children, even if they have apparently made a full recovery. Educational or behavioural difficulties may not be present until the child is fully reintegrated back at home and school. Difficulties in some of the higher mental functions, including processing and perception, may be quite subtle; the same applies to problems with attention and concentration which may, not infrequently, become apparent when the child is back in school and being stretched. This can result in learning difficulties which, if not recognized, may ultimately present as a behaviour problem.

Unfortunately, not all teachers or educational psychologists have the expertise to identify these often subtle learning difficulties or realize their significance. The community paediatrician who has established links with the school is able to alert teachers and psychologists of such potential difficulties in order that they may be anticipated, promptly recognized, and fully assessed.

Finally, the community paediatrician will, of course, seek expert advice from members of the rehabilitation team, should this be necessary.

Behaviour problems associated with brain injury have been described in Chapter 9. Their severity may not become apparent until the child is back in his community. It then can become obvious the child 'has changed'. Pupils, teachers, and parents frequently find this difficult to cope with and are unsure how to handle such problems. Often, children are simply labelled as being 'naughty' and, consequently, disciplined, which merely exacerbates the problem. Unless the child is followed up this may not come to the attention of the professionals until he is excluded or the parents are no longer able to cope with his difficult behaviour.

Close working with schools, the educational psychologist, and child and adolescent mental health service is essential to identify – and manage – the problem successfully. Again, it is usually the community paediatrician who is the most suitable person to ensure that the relevant professionals are involved at the appropriate time.

Ongoing advice to the local education authority

The statutory responsibility that community doctors have to notify the education authority of a child who may have special educational needs and to contribute to the assessment has already been discussed. Educational assessment may be necessary at any stage following discharge; because of this the community paediatrician will need to be kept up to date with every aspect of the child's physical, cognitive, and emotional status in order that they can contribute meaningfully to the educational assessment.

Annual review of a child with a statement of educational needs has been formalized under the 1993 Education Act. Where there are health needs, the community paediatrician and therapists will be asked to submit a report for the review of the child's progress and also to attend the review if possible. It is very important that childrens' health needs are adequately catered for in school so that they can realize their maximum potential. It is essential that the school doctor ensures that all relevant information is made available to the school.

School doctors should also ensure that information on the child's school progress, and any concerns that the teacher may have regarding the child's health or emotional development, is fed back to hospital specialists. Children spend a considerable number of hours in school per week and teaching staff are in an ideal position to detect any changes in the physical and emotional well-being of the child. Feedback from schools is particularly important in the diagnosis and subsequent management of epilepsy. It is not uncommon for teachers to be the first to raise concerns because of a fall-off in school performance which they would not expect, and one cause for this decline in performance may be the development of epilepsy, particularly complex partial seizures.

Confidentiality is, of course, important. Obtaining permission to share information with other professionals rarely poses a problem, particularly if doctors have always worked closely and openly with parents.

Support for the family

There will need to be considerable input for children who have residual problems. However, even if the child has made a full recovery the family may still need support. Are parents who have almost lost a child able to treat that child the same as before? Are parents more likely to indulge them and be less strict with them than before? If so, siblings can often feel resentful. The child himself may find it difficult to return to the normality of home and school and cease being the centre of attention. School may exacerbate this situation by continuing to treat the child as special, and both schoolteachers and parents can often overprotect the child sometimes without realizing it. Regular review by the community paediatrician can assist parents to help their child reintegrate back into home and school life. They can ensure that the school is acting appropriately and offer advice as required. Such advice and guidance may help to prevent the development of serious behaviour problems.

Advocacy is an important role of the community paediatrician. This may take many forms, ranging from advocacy for an individual child to advocacy at national and international levels. Resources are scarce within health, social services, and education and many parents of disabled children have to assume the fighter or 'terrier' role to achieve and secure adequate services for their children. Understandably, not all parents are able, or feel comfortable adopting this (at times) relatively aggressive approach. When it is clear that a child is not receiving appropriate services then the community paediatrician can frequently offer support and advice to parents on how to best express their concerns with the different agencies and authorities.

SUMMARY

Brain injury is a traumatic event and experience for the child, family, and friends. The child may make a full recovery or be left with varying degrees of different disabilities. Whatever the outcome, the child will return to his community where he has the right to receive the necessary and appropriate schooling and care to help achieve his maximal potential – physically, emotionally, socially and cognitively. The hospital rehabilitation team must work and liaise closely with the professionals in the community who, ultimately will be responsible for ongoing support in order to achieve this objective.

REFERENCES

Bax, M.C.O. and Whitmore, K. (1991). District handicap teams in England: 1983–8. *Archives of Disease in Childhood*, **66**, 656–64.

British Paediatric Association. (1991). *Towards a combined child health service*. BPA, London.

British Paediatric Association. (1992). *Community child health services; an information base for purchasers*. BPA, London.

Court Report. (1976). *Fit for the future: The report of the Committee on Child Health Services*. Chairman: S.D.M. Court. HMSO, London.

Department of Education. (1994). *Code of practice (for the implementation of the 1993 Education Act)*. HMSO, London.

Duckworth, G. (1990). Revised guidelines for the control of epidemic methicillin-resistant *staphylococcus aureus*. Working party report. *Journal of Hospital Infection* **16**, 351–77.

Polnay, L. (1995). *Health needs of school age children*. Report of a joint working party. Chairman: L. Polnay. BPA, London.

11

The impact of brain injury on the family

Colin Demellweek and Audrey O'Leary

INTRODUCTION

When a child suffers a brain injury (BI), other family members are likely to be affected and, indeed, such an injury has been referred to as being a family affair (Lezak 1988). Family members may be there when the injury occurs or be called to the hospital afterwards, and even quite a mild head injury (HI) appears to cause parents anxiety. In more severe cases, the child may be in a coma and family members may spend long, uncertain hours at the child's bedside, disrupting family routines. If and when the child emerges from the coma he may, for example, be unable to walk or talk. A lengthy rehabilitation process may then begin, again requiring family members to spend long periods of time in the hospital and suspend or defer other activities. Rehabilitation may only be partly successful in alleviating deficits due to the BI and a very different child may rejoin the family, following discharge. In particular, the child is likely to have more emotional, behavioural, and social problems than before the injury (see Chapter 9). The psychological adjustment of individual family members and the way in which the family functions as a whole may, therefore, be impaired. Any such impairment is not only of intrinsic importance but also has implications for the post-injury adjustment of the brain-injured child. Depressed parents, for instance, tend to be inconsistent in their interactions with children and brain-injured children often need very consistent management.

Methodological and other issues

Although having a child suffer a brain injury would be expected to affect other family members, there is a paucity of research into this issue. As a consequence, it is necessary to draw on research with adults with BI and children with chronic illness and congenital disabilities. Findings from these areas of research which appear, clinically, to be particularly relevant to paediatric brain injury will, therefore, be referred to. There are, however, a number of methodological issues which should be borne in mind when evaluating the studies to be described (Brooks 1991; Wade *et al.* 1995). First, difficulties observed following brain injury may have existed prior to the injury being sustained. Second, some problems family members are found to have post-injury may be related to having had a child suffer an injury rather than a brain injury in particular. Third, the stresses and strains the family may face may change over time and so, therefore, may family adjustment (Ponsford 1995).

Effect on parents

That the psychological adjustment of carers of adults with BI can be impaired is well-established (Brooks 1991). In one study (Kreutzer *et al.* 1994), such carers were assessed 1.5 to 60 months (mean = 16 months) after the injury and 47% were sufficiently distressed to warrant clinical intervention. Levels of anxiety, depression, hostility, and somaticization were particularly elevated. Also common were feelings of isolation and of being alienated from others together with feelings of burden, responsibility, and of being overwhelmed. In carers of adult BI survivors, levels of anxiety and depression may fluctuate with time but can remain elevated for many years (Brooks 1991). It is also well-established that having a child suffer a chronic illness (Eiser 1993) or congenital physical disability (Beresford 1994) puts parents at risk of developing psychological problems. In addition, maternal psychological adjustment appears to be affected following general paediatric traumatic injuries (see Wade *et al.* 1995). In one study, children admitted to a paediatric trauma centre because of severe injury (including but not restricted to HI) were followed up for a year. Rates of maternal psychological disorder increased markedly from premorbid (i.e. pre-injury) levels of 16% to about 59% whilst the child was in hospital and declined slowly over the following year to about 41%. Preliminary evidence suggests that the level of maternal psychological distress is higher after a child has suffered a moderate to severe HI compared to an orthopaedic injury (Taylor *et al.* 1995).

Siblings

Although considerable concern has been expressed about the effect on siblings of having a brother or sister suffer a BI (Waaland and Kreutzer 1988), there appears to have been only one formal (and small) study of this particular issue (Orsillo *et al.* 1993). The results of this study suggest that such concern is justified since 10 of 12 siblings (83%) assessed 1 – 149 months post-injury, had levels of psychological distress sufficient to warrant clinical intervention. The pattern of distress exhibited by the siblings appears to have been similar to that shown by carers of adults with BI discussed previously, such as feelings of alienation. In another, largely subjective, study (see Wade *et al.* 1995), parents of children admitted to a paediatric trauma centre (some of whom had been admitted because of head injuries) were interviewed at least 1 year after discharge. Parents reported that 46% of the uninjured siblings had developed some emotional reactions, school problems, or aggressive personality problems.

Although these latter two studies have methodological limitations, their findings are consistent with research into the effects on siblings of having a child with chronic illness in the family (Eiser 1993). Such siblings can experience frequent separations from their parents, have their daily routines disrupted, have less chance to relax and interact with their parents, and can easily be overlooked by medical staff and parents. As a consequence, jealousy, hostility, and aggression may be shown towards the ill child but siblings may also feel guilty for doing so. Siblings of brain-injured children are likely to have similar experiences and so have similar reactions to the injured child. In addition, they may be given more responsibility within the home and, because their brother or sister has lost friends (see Chapter 9), be expected to provide him or her with company. Furthermore, the injured child faced with peer ridicule and academic failure can redirect feelings of anger and frustration toward family members (Waaland and Kreutzer 1988). Moreover, poor parental mental health and impaired family functioning would be expected to affect the adjustment of all the children in the family. Whether or not siblings develop problems is, however, likely to depend on a number of factors such as their age, temperament, and the availability of support (for example, from extended family members and friends).

Although evidence suggests that the relationship between brain-injured children and their siblings deteriorates following the injury (Rivara *et al.* 1992), siblings can also be quite protective of, and concerned about, the injured child.

Effects on the family as a unit

In families, roles evolve for individual members as do rules to live by, communication patterns, and ways to solve problems and negotiate with each other, all of which can be disrupted when a family member suffers a BI (DePompei and Williams 1994). Consistent with this suggestion, impaired post-injury family functioning has been reported by parents (Bragg *et al.* 1992) and siblings (Orsillo et al, 1993) of brain-injured children. Unhealthy, post-injury functioning was also reported by 56% of carers of adults with BI in one study (Kreutzer *et al.* 1994).

Although pre-injury functioning appears to be the best predictor of family functioning following BI, such functioning does appear to deteriorate following the injury (Taylor *et al.* 1995), particularly if it has been severe (Rivara *et al.* 1992). The marital relationship may deteriorate and parents of children with moderate to severe BI report having more family disagreements than do parents of children with orthopaedic injuries (Taylor *et al*. 1995).

Although there are disagreements about key concepts and definitions of family functioning, aspects which may be affected (Kreutzer *et al*. 1994) include:

- the family's ability to resolve problems
- the efficacy with which tasks (practical and emotional) are allocated and accomplished within the family
- the ability of members to respond to each other in an appropriate emotional manner
- the quality of interest, concern, and investment family members have for each other
- the standards and latitudes that are set for behaviour within the family
- the effectiveness, extent, clarity, and directness with which information is exchanged within the family.

FACTORS INFLUENCING FAMILY ADJUSTMENT

Although the adjustment of individual family members and the family as a unit may be affected when a child suffers a BI, it is clear that many families cope very well. This also seems to be the case when a child in the family has a chronic illness (Eiser, 1993) or congenital disability (Beresford 1994), findings which have led to attempts to identify factors which influence adjustment. A model has been put forward to account for differences in family adjustment after a child has, specifically, suffered a BI (Wade *et al*. 1995) which is shown in Fig. 11.1. In this model, family adaptation is seen as being 'a function of a complex transaction amongst injury sequelae and burden, family resources, and the broader environmental context' (Wade *et al*. 1995, p747).

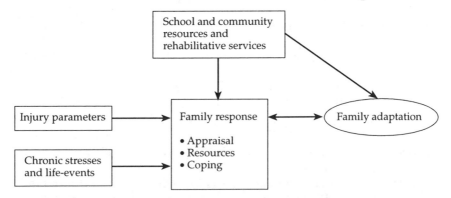

Fig. 11.1 Framework of factors influencing family adaptation following traumatic brain injury. (Reproduced with permission from Wade *et al*. (1995). *Journal of Pediatric Psychology*, Plenum Publishing Corporation.)

Injury parameters

In terms of injury parameters, stress may stem from medical management, disruption of family routines, concerns with spouse and siblings, and concerns about the future. The financial cost to the family when a child suffers a BI can also be considerable. The cost of rehabilitation services in the USA can be very high and may not be covered completely by private insurance (Brooks 1991). In the UK, rehabilitation services (if available) are usually provided by the National Health Service. Parents may, however, have to cease work to care for the brain-injured child, resulting in a loss of income. There may also be additional costs in terms of transport (for hospital appointments, etc.) and items of equipment needed by the injured child. Other potential sources of stress are detailed below.

Contact with health, social, and educational professionals

Having a child suffer a BI can bring the family into contact with a large number of such professionals. Obviously, staff are there to help the brain injured child and his family, however, the potential stressfulness of this contact should not be underestimated . Mothers of children with congenital disabilities can report finding such involvement stressful (Beresford 1994), whilst learning to be assertive with professionals has been reported by wives of men with BI as being a valuable skill to develop (see Ponsford 1995).

Acquisition of knowledge relevant to brain injury

Although parents usually have a great thirst for such information, their existing knowledge, particularly concerning prognosis, is likely to be poor. For example, many adults do not appear to know the size and position of the brain within the skull. The complexity of the information family members may need to assimilate, for instance concerning the nature of executive dysfunction (see Chapter 9), also needs to be recognized. Terms routinely used by staff, such as hemiplegia, hemianopia, apraxia, and ataxia are unlikely to be familiar to the family whilst terms like pre-morbid may be frightening. One mother has reported that when she first heard this latter term being applied to her son she thought staff may have been predicting his death (Williams and Kay 1991). Parents may also have to learn about the complex rules governing educational provision and welfare benefits for children with BI (see Chapters 8 and 10).

Involvement with the legal system

For some families, having a child suffer a brain injury involves them in legal proceedings, which was identified in one small study as being amongst the five most pressing problems faced by mothers of adolescents and young men with BI (see Ponsford 1995). In the UK, an adversarial system operates in which compensation is awarded on the basis of proven responsibility (decided on the basis of probability) coupled with the extent of the brain-injury survivors impairment. In some cases, legal proceedings are protracted and bring survivor's and their families into contact with yet more professionals, including lawyers and possibly specialists in accident reconstruction. Parents may have to sit and listen to the circumstances of the accident being discussed objectively, which can be very distressing. Often, repeated assessments are carried out and parents may have to reiterate the history of the accident and subsequent effect on the child and themselves many times. Compensation can involve large sums of money and parents can feel that they are being accused of 'cheating' or of being 'gold-diggers'. Parents may, therefore, need to be reassured of the legal and moral right of children injured through no fault of their own to compensation. Some carers begin to worry how the brain-injured child would cope if anything happened to them and appropriate monetary compensation can sometimes ease their fears.

Changes to the brain-injured child

In the long term, it is the changes to the child caused by the BI which are likely to be the greatest cause of stress for family members. For the carers of adults with BI the changes in the survivor's emotional control, behaviour, and personality are the major sources of subjective feelings of burden (Brooks 1991) and equate most strongly with the carer's mental health (Kreutzer *et al.* 1994). In children with Down's syndrome, the child's behaviour problems are strongly related to maternal self-reported psychological distress (Beresford 1994). Parents of brain-injured children report finding the parenting of these children more stressful than the parenting of their siblings (Perrot *et al* 1991). Sequelae of BI such as emotional disinhibition, difficulty learning from experience, and impulsivity require parents to change expectations, rules, and disciplinary practices (Lezak 1988). Changes to children, following HI, which have been found to cause parents moderate to severe strain one year post injury include their difficulty remembering the right word, temper outbursts, irritability, distractibility, difficulty following things through, lack of initiative, need for supervision, forgetfulness, and personality changes (Rivara *et al.* 1992).

Chronic stresses and life-events

As well as stress arising from the child's injury, other chronic stresses and life-events may be important in determining family adjustment and tip the balance against successful adaptation. Thus, a family may cope well following the child's brain injury until a parent is made redundant from work. Some families may be struggling with such stressors even before the child suffers the injury. In one study (Rivara *et al.* 1992), a greater than expected percentage of families (compared to population norms) had, prior to the child's HI, experienced; intrafamily problems, illness and family care strains, and work and family changes.

Family response

Although having a child suffer a brain injury is likely to expose the family to a variety of potential stressors, the way in which the family members deal with such stressors and the resources at their disposal are likely to be important in determining adjustment.

Appraisal

Appraisal refers to the perception, interpretation, and cognitive representation of events by individuals. Such appraisal, particularly of injury parameters, is likely to affect adjustment following a child's brain injury. For example, families frequently seem to appraise the extent to which the accident was preventable, which is related to assessments of guilt and blame. Failure to resolve this issue may affect coping and impede transition from the crisis phase following the injury (Wade *et al.* 1995).

Most accidents, with hindsight, could have been prevented, often by having had the child stay at home on that particular day. It is also sometimes possible to identify someone who can be blamed for the injury. This may, for instance, be the child (e.g. for not taking sufficient care crossing the road) or the driver of a car. Parents may also blame themselves, for example, for buying the child the bike he was riding in the accident. It seems natural for parents to want to consider and discuss this issue, and work out what could be done in the future to prevent a further injury. Some parents, however, appear to get stuck on this issue and perhaps resort to 'wishful thinking' (e.g. 'If only I hadn't let him go out that day') which may impair their ability to deal with the consequences of the injury.

Families also tend to appraise the degree to which the child has recovered or will do so in the future and the extent of the child's emotional motivation. This latter assessment can be particularly important to adaptation if slow progress is seen as being due to a lack of motivation rather than other factors (Wade *et al.* 1995). In addition, appraisal of the significance of the consequences of the brain injury may be important. For instance, in families where high value is placed on academic achievement, a child's loss of academic abilities may be particularly distressing.

Resources

Family resources include the characteristics of individual family members, such as education, physical health, and psychological adjustment. For example, more highly educated parents are likely to find it easier to assimilate and understand information concerning the effects of the injury. Parents' personality characteristics may be particularly important in adaptation. High scores on the neuroticism scale (a measure of emotionality) of the Eysenck Personality Inventory (EPI) are associated with reports of high levels of burden by the carers of adults with BI (Brooks 1991) and poor psychological adjustment in mothers of children with Down's syndrome (Beresford 1994).

The importance of extraversion in parental adaptation is, however, less clear. Scores on this scale of the EPI do not appear to be related to carers' subjective reports of burden, following BI to adults (Brooks 1991). Extraversion is, however, linked to maternal adaptation to, and acceptance of, congenitally physically-disabled children (Beresford 1994). Clinically, it seems that extroverts are better able to cope with brain-injured children. For instance, as many as 40% of adults with BI have been reported by carers as showing inappropriate public behaviour. Extroverts may be better able to cope with the attention such behaviour attracts, and contact with professionals, than do introverts.

Family resources also include the characteristics of the family as a unit (such as adaptability, cohesion, organization, communication, and religious values) along with other resources such as the availability of social support. Family cohesiveness may be particularly important in adaptation, especially when it becomes clear that the child's deficits are likely to be permanent. Enmeshed families (i.e. those showing excessive togetherness, lack of privacy for individuals, and intrusiveness) may be prone to depression and prolonged mourning, whilst disengaged families (i.e. those with an exaggerated sense of the independence of individuals and where high stress is needed to activate intrafamily support systems) may become angry, frustrated, and resentful (Rape *et al.* 1992).

The practical resources available to the family are also likely to be important in adjustment. Thus, car ownership is significantly related to the psychological adjustment of mothers of children with Down's syndrome (Beresford 1994) and is likely to influence parental levels of stress after a child has had a BI. Using public transport with a child who has a physical disability or disinhibited behaviour poses considerable problems.

Coping

It is well-established that coping strategies are related to the adjustment of parents of chronically ill (Eiser 1993) and physically disabled children

(Beresford 1994). Although there are a number of ways in which coping strategies can be conceptualized, a commonly made distinction is between what can be called problem- and emotion-focused coping (see Beresford 1994). Problem-focused coping involves attempts to change aspects of the person or environment (or the relationship between these two elements) which is seen as being stressful. Thus, following BI, a child may be hyperactive. An example of problem-focused coping in relation to this behaviour would be to reduce the number of distractions in the environment so as to reduce the child's activity levels. Emotion-focused coping strategies, on the other hand, involve attempts to manage or regulate negative emotions associated with the stressor. These include denial/avoidance, distraction/minimization, wishful thinking, self-control of feelings, seeking meaning, self-blame, and expressing/sharing feelings, among other strategies. Research in paediatric populations suggests that problem-focused coping is associated with better outcome (Eiser 1993). Emotion-focused coping may, however, be helpful with less controllable stressors (Beresford 1994). Usefulness may also depend on the type of emotion-focused coping strategy employed. For instance, positively reframing a problem may be an effective strategy in reducing stress, whilst husbands of brain-injured wives report that maintaining a sense of humour is an important coping strategy (see Ponsford 1995). Wishful thinking, however, is generally associated with poor adjustment (Beresford 1994).

Rehabilitative services and resources available in the school and community

The family response and adaptation is also likely to be influenced by resources available at school and in the community. In this light it is important to note that there are concerns about the ability of schools in the UK and in the USA to deal with brain-injured children (Savage and Carter, in Williams and Kay 1991). Rehabilitative services are obviously important for helping a child recover as much ability as possible and so minimize stress from injury parameters but are also important in other ways. For example, education about executive dysfunction may influence appraisal of the child's behaviour so that it is not simply seen as being naughtiness or due to lack of motivation.

INTERVENTIONS

Given the stress the family is placed under when a child has a BI, it is likely that many families would benefit from psychological help. Interventions will obviously be based on assessment of factors such as those outlined in the model discussed previously, but it has been suggested that there are three levels at which such help can be provided (Kay and Cavello, 1994). These are:

(1) information and education
(2) support, problem solving, and restructuring
(3) formal therapy.

Six forms which family intervention can take have also been identified (Muir *et al.* 1990). These are:

(1) patient–family education;
(2) family therapy;
(3) family counselling;
(4) behavioural family training;
(5) respite care;
(6) family support groups.

Behavioural management is outlined in Chapter 9 and so will not be reiterated here. Respite care appears to be effective in helping parents of children with congenital physical disabilities cope (see Beresford 1994) and is likely to be of benefit to some parents of brain-injured children.

As well as intervention being possible at different levels, there can be three different targets for interventions (Kay and Cavello 1994). First, there are individual family members. Thus, one parent may be having particular difficulty dealing with the child's injury because, for example, of unresolved issues relating to a previous loss such as the death of a parent. Second, there is the family system. Third, there is the relationship between the family and the wider community, both social and professional. Of particular importance within the professional community is the rehabilitation team and the school (Kay and Cavello 1994). The team needs to understand strongly-held family norms and values if impasse in the rehabilitation process is to be avoided. Similarly, as will be discussed later, the relationship the family has with the child's school is crucial and will frequently need to be addressed.

Help can be given at three stages following BI, these being acute care, rehabilitation, and community reintegration. The sort of help the family needs, and equally importantly, will accept, is likely, however, to change over time and so possible interventions will be considered in detail in terms of these stages following the injury.

Acute phase

When a child is first admitted to hospital following a brain injury, the parental response is usually one of shock – accidents, by their nature, being unpredictable. Most head injuries are mild and the hospital stay might brief, although still anxiety-provoking. More severe injuries may, however, require neurosurgical intervention and possible admission to an intensive-care unit (ICU). Besides the obvious fear of death, the three main sources of stress for parents of critically ill children appear to be the sights and sounds of the unit, the child's physical appearance and behaviour, and parental role alterations, i.e. from being the primary carers for the child, parents are largely reduced to the role of spectator. Parents seem to focus very much on the needs of the injured child at this time and see their own needs as being relatively unimportant (see Kepler, in Singer *et al.* 1996).

Provision of information

Parents of brain-injured children stress the importance of being given straightforward, timely, and honest information about the child's condition and progress, and may vividly remember some things they are told in the acute phase which can influence their reaction to subsequent information. Thus, parents who are told their child will never walk may lose faith in professionals if this does not turn out to be the case. For this reason it has been suggested that absolutes such as 'never' or 'complete' are not used and that the term 'improvement' is preferable to 'recovery'. A clear, under-standable explanation of the name and function of the equipment being used should also be provided. Misinterpretations, for example of the child's body movements, should also be corrected without removing a sense of hope (Rivara 1994). Although many parents appear to cope well with the confusional state which can occur as the child emerges from a coma, some may be embarrassed by behaviour such as swearing or lashing out at staff. Parents may need to be reassured that such behaviour is normal and not a reflection of their parenting abilities. It is also important, however, that parents and staff do not reinforce such behaviour in their pleasure at the child's emergence from the coma.

Involvement of parents

As the critical role in the child's life is occupied by medical and nursing staff, at this stage parents may have strong feelings of helplessness, which, if continued, may affect parental confidence in the future. Assigning appro-priate tasks to parents may increase their sense of competence (Rivara 1994). Once it is clear that the child will live, parents obviously experience considerable relief. He may, however, only slowly emerge from the coma, in which case the parents may spend long hours trying to stimulate him via strategies such as attempting to get the child's favourite pop or football star to visit or provide a tape-recording. Such strategies may well be worth trying and may reduce carers' feelings of helplessness. It is, however, important to ensure there are no feelings of guilt if they are not effective (Ponsford 1995).

Provision of support

In the early stages following a BI, friends and family appear to rally round and provide parents with their main source of emotional support. Physicians, nurses, and social workers may also provide such support. Parents appear to look very much to each other for support and single parents may, therefore, be particularly vulnerable and more in need of professional help. Parents do not seem to want to meet parents of other children in the same position for group discussions (see Kepler, in Singer *et al.* 1996). In some circumstances, however, they may benefit from being introduced, individually or as a couple, to other parents whose child suffered a similar injury in the past and who can provide a model of successful coping. Although feelings of anxiety and depression are understandable, parents who react particularly strongly in this stage may be at risk for future problems and so may require early intervention.

   Parents may be largely limited to using emotion-focused coping strategies (other than information-seeking) when the child is first in a coma. A variety of strategies may be used, such as turning to religion or trying to find meaning in the situation. Self-blame may also occur, however, in which case parents may need to be reminded that their intentions are good and it is not possible to protect children absolutely (Rivara 1994). Clinical experience suggests that mothers and fathers tend to use different coping strategies, with men being more likely to use denial or suppression of feelings than women.

Appointment of an advocate

It has been recommended that an advocate be appointed to liaise between the family and medical, nursing, and therapy staff. The role of the advocate is to provide the family with clear, understandable information concerning the patient and to make staff aware of the family's concerns. This is not intended to preclude contact between the family and these professionals but acknowledges their workload and the family's likely need for information to be given repeatedly if it is to be comprehended and understood (Ponsford 1995). Given the possible need of the family for practical and financial help, it is likely, and important, that a social worker makes contact with the family soon after the child's admission, and so may be ideally placed to take on the role of an advocate. Having established a relationship with the family, it is likely to be beneficial if the social worker could continue to offer support throughout the rehabilitation process and beyond (Ponsford 1995). As the transfer of the child to a rehabilitation unit nears, it would seem good practice for the parents to visit the unit and be introduced to the staff there by the advocate/social worker.

Needs of siblings

Siblings of the brain-injured child may fare particularly badly in the acute phase as the parents focus very much on the needs of the ill child and in the acquisition of knowledge about his condition and progress. Parents ensure that siblings are physically cared for, but their psychological needs may go unnoticed as the parents struggle to cope with the situation. In particular, siblings' need for information about the ill child may go unmet. Parents may, however, need advice about how to respond to siblings' questions (Rivara 1994).

Rehabilitation phase

The time a child spends in a rehabilitation unit can vary considerably, depending on a number of factors such as the severity of the injury, resources available in the unit and (particularly in the USA) financial factors. Although for most children this period is usually short (a few days to a week or so), it may be prolonged and can continue for many weeks or even months.

Contact with rehabilitation professionals

Admission to the rehabilitation unit brings parents into contact with a large number of new professionals. As well as a new set of medical and nursing staff, there are numerous others who will be involved in the child's rehabilitation. Whilst parents will be familiar with the teacher's and possibly physiotherapist's roles, it is less likely that they will know what other professionals do. It is important, therefore, that staff *repeatedly* introduce themselves to the parents and explain their role. Written material can be provided which outlines the role of various professionals. In the UK, the Children's Head Injury Trust (CHIT) provides such material, or the unit may produce its own, as we do at Alder Hey. Given the number of professionals involved in rehabilitating the child, the need for a family advocate/social worker to liaise between staff and the family is likely to continue.

Education

It is during the rehabilitation phase that parents may acquire much of their understanding about the nature and consequences of brain injury. Topics of interest may include mechanisms of brain injury, management of coma and post-traumatic amnesia (PTA), medical complications (e.g. epilepsy and diabetes insipidus), the nature and management of various disorders (mobility, communication, swallowing, cognition, behaviour, and emotion), accessing community resources, and financial and legal issues (Ponsford 1995). These informational needs may be met in support groups, which are discussed later. In the absence of such groups, rehabilitation staff may need to provide such information individually. A number of books about brain injury have also been written for family members in general (Deaton 1987; Gronwall *et al.* 1990) and children in particular (Raines and Waaland 1992), which can supplement information given verbally.

Involvement of parents in rehabilitation

The importance of involving the family in rehabilitation has been repeatedly stressed (DePompei and Williams 1994; Rivara 1994) and parents often express a wish to be treated as partners rather than patients. Parents can become involved in setting rehabilitation goals and providing information about the child which can be used in choosing rewards or making therapy more meaningful to him (DePompei and Williams, 1994). Simply having parents sit in on sessions may alleviate the child's anxiety which, it is well-established, can impede learning. Parents can also take a more active role in teaching the child skills and may acquire knowledge, such as task analysis, which they can use when the child returns home. Involvement in rehabilitation sessions may also make the child's difficulties more clear to parents, making it less likely that denial will occur. Such involvement may also make it less likely that learned helplessness will develop in parents, something which is of concern following BI (Brooks 1991), and it has been argued that parents should only be excluded from rehabilitation sessions if they are disruptive (DePompei and Williams 1994).

Having siblings sit in on sessions may help them see that being in a rehabilitation unit is hard work for the child, and so possibly assuage feelings of resentment.

Parents may, however, also become overinvolved in rehabilitation to the detriment of their own needs and those of other family members. Parents may need to be given permission, or indeed encouraged, to spend less time in the unit, provided they are comfortable about doing so (Ponsford 1995), and gently reminded of the needs of siblings (Rivara 1994).

Support groups

It is often in this phase that families may join a support group if one is available. At a broad level, the goal of such groups is to meet the educational and emotional needs of the members (see Williams, in Singer *et al.* 1996 for a full discussion of support groups). Groups often have a speaker on a particular topic, such as those described previously, followed by a group discussion. A particularly important aspect of such groups may be to reduce families' social isolation, which often appears to occur after a member has had a BI. Bonds formed between members at this time may be important once rehabilitation support ceases and support from friends and family diminishes (Ponsford 1995).

Although an aim of support groups may be to allow members to discuss their own emotional reactions to the injury and sequelae, participants' willingness to do so is likely to depend on the time since the injury and the stage of the family's adjustment. Parents may be unwilling to discuss their own emotions initially but concentrate very much on their child's needs. If carers are to discuss their own emotional reactions and needs it is important that suitably trained rehabilitation professionals take a facilitative or guiding role and that some issues are taken up individually (Ponsford 1995). Again, this facilitative role is most likely to be taken by a family advocate/social worker.

Although the potential benefits of support groups can be considerable, the maintenance of such groups can be problematic. Group membership tends to fluctuate and appears to depend on a number of factors, including location, the distance participants have to travel, and the availability of parking and child-care facilities. New members appear to need the support of veterans if regular participation is to be achieved. Unfortunately, the issues which veterans may wish to discuss may be different to those of new members, resulting in a decline in attendance. Possible benefits of membership of support groups include improved relationships with extended family members, enhanced confidence about decision making abilities (particularly in relation to educational provision for the BI child), and the solution of conflicts with school personnel. It appears that siblings rarely attend such support groups and the form meetings take (i.e. heavily based on discussion) may, indeed, be inappropriate for younger children. Siblings may, therefore, need to take part in simulated rehabilitation sessions, followed by discussions, if they are to understand the changes in their brother or sister and the process of rehabilitation.

Mobilizing social support

Families of BI survivors may become increasingly isolated socially following discharge (Lezak 1988) because, for example, of embarrassment at the survivor's behaviour, or others tiring of hearing about the injury. Given the value of social support, it would seem important to try to prevent such isolation occurring, and a social-network intervention for mobilizing social support has been described (Rogers and Kreutzer 1984). This intervention involves gathering together immediate family members along with extended family, friends, and acquaintances. Participants are informed about the effects of the injury and likely outcome, potential problems and solutions are generated, goals are formulated, and individual responsibilities identified. Further sessions are held to provide participants with new information concerning the BI survivor and monitor progress towards, and, if necessary, alter, goals. Although there can be considerable practical difficulties in arranging sessions, the intervention may result in networks sharing the burden and, importantly, averting future crises.

Liaison with local services

Towards the end of the intensive rehabilitation it will have become clearer which of the child's deficits are likely to be prolonged, if not permanent. Contact will therefore need to be made with local social services concerning the child's needs for adaption to, and equipment for, the home. Such needs are likely to have been identified during his visits home prior to discharge.

Dealing with denial

The child's admission to the rehabilitation unit often appears to herald a period of optimism for the family (Rivara 1994). Initially, improvement, particularly in terms of physical abilities, may be quite rapid, thereby fostering feelings of hope. Family members can therefore become frustrated when and if progress slows, and the consequent feelings may be directed at rehabilitation staff and need to be handled tactfully (Ponsford 1995). Family members may also deny any deficits or difficulties exhibited by the brain-injured child. The issue of denial is complex, however, (Deaton 1986), and it appears to be more likely to occur in relation to the child's cognitive and behavioural difficulties than his motor deficits.

Denial may also take different forms. Pre-morbid skills may be under-estimated and a child may, for example, be described as never having talked much. Signs of improvement that do not really exist may also be seen by parents. Thus, vocalizations may be interpreted as words rather than sounds. Parents may also overestimate the degree and rate of improvement that is possible, such as the parents who expect a child with a severe BI to sit an examination in a few weeks' time. Many people's ideas about brain injury may be based on depictions in television in which periods of unconsciousness are followed by few, if any, lasting effects. Not surprisingly, therefore, parents' hopes of recovery may be high, and in some instances denial may reflect a lack of knowledge rather than a psychological defence. When it does do so, however, it may prevent parents being overwhelmed by the changes to their child and the implications that these changes can have for their own lives (Kay and Cavello 1994) thus allowing the reality of the injury to be gradually absorbed (Martin 1988).

Denial may also have a positive influence on the child's recovery. Thus, setting the child goals which appear at first sight to be over-optimistic may result in the achievement of these goals (Deaton 1986). There may, however, also be disadvantages of denial. Children may be set over-optimistic goals that, when they are not achieved, cause feelings of failure and even despair. Parents who deny deficits may accuse children of not trying hard enough (Wade *et al.* 1995), whilst parents who refuse to accept the limitations of treatment may go 'doctor shopping' (Brooks 1991), requesting second and third (or more) medical opinions. Denial becomes problematic if it is prolonged, treatments necessary for improvement are refused, or a family member is in some way endangered (DePompei and Williams 1994).

The question of how to deal with denial has been subject to considerable discussion (Deaton 1986) but little empirical investigation. There does, however, seem to be a consensus that denial should be respected, the positive elements recognized, and that direct confrontation is largely ineffective. Repeated confrontation can result in the alienation of the family which may then be difficult to overcome (Ponsford 1995). It has been argued that individuals who have had a brain injury should be slowly, carefully, and respectfully shown their limitations (see Chapter 9). This approach may also be effective with family members. They could, for example, sit in on a session designed to evaluate a child's understanding of language, in which the availability of visual clues is systematically varied. From this it follows that denial may be less likely to occur (or be less extreme) if parents are involved in rehabilitation sessions from an early stage.

Return to school

Although the child's discharge from in-patient rehabilitation may be considered to be the start of the community reintegration phase, the child's return to school can pose particular problems for the parents and will, therefore, be considered separately. The return to school is taken by many brain-injured children and their families to indicate a return to normality, but this need not necessarily be the case and, instead, a new set of potential stressors may have to be faced (see Glang *et al.*, in Singer *et al* [1996] for a full discussion of the difficulties parents may encounter).

Support for parents

The rules governing the provision of education for children with special educational needs (as can follow a brain injury) are quite complex. Although written material may be available to explain the procedures to be followed, parents may still need to be guided through them. In addition, brain-injured children may not fit easily into existing special educational categories. As a consequence, parents may have much more contact with education personnel than is usual and they may find this contact stressful.

Parents also often have to deal with the psychological reaction of the child following his return to school. Children moving to a 'special' school can blame parents for the placement, possibly stimulating feelings of guilt and failure on their part. At the same time, of course, parents may be struggling with their own feelings of loss triggered by the move. For the brain-injured child returning to his previous school, the picture may be somewhat different. As noted in Chapter 9, his self-esteem may gradually erode as difficulties become more clear and academic progress is slowed. Parents have to try to support their child when this occurs and perhaps also deal with his reaction to being teased or taken advantage of by peers. It is often very difficult for parents to cope with their child's resulting distress.

Liaison with the school

There is obviously a need for rehabilitation staff to liaise with the brain-injured child's school concerning his educational needs and this issue has been addressed in Chapter 10. There is also, however, a need for liaison to occur in relation to the child's emotional, behaviourial, and social difficulties. As brain-injured children often make a good physical recovery, the unwarranted assumption may be made that a good recovery has been made in other areas. Furthermore, teachers' knowledge of the consequences of BI is often minimal and clinical experience suggests that their knowledge of the behavioural, emotional, and social difficulties which can follow BI is particularly limited (see Savage and Carter, in Williams and Kay 1991). As a result, unrealistic expectations may be held about the child. It is important, therefore, that school staff are provided with information relating to this issue. In particular, school staff need to be given information concerning any executive function deficits the child has, otherwise there is a danger that the child will be labelled 'naughty', which may in turn be attributed to poor parenting practices. For example, perseveration may be labelled 'stubbornness' and difficulties in processing socio-emotional information (see Chapter 9) attributed to rudeness. Even with such liaison, labelling may still occur, particularly if the child had pre-injury problems, and this may be difficult to overcome.

Community reintegration

Following discharge from rehabilitation, the child and his family have to try to re-enter community life, often having had their circumstances radically altered, and it is at that point that the emotional impact of the injury is most likely to be felt (Kay and Cavello 1994). As a consequence, it is at this time that formal psychological help is most needed and most requested.

Stage models of family adaptation

It has been argued that when an individual suffers a brain injury, the family response can be characterized in terms of psychological phases or stages. A number of different models have been put forward (see Rape *et al.* 1992) but the following stages are commonly referred to:

- shock
- relief, denial, and unrealistic expectations
- emotional turmoil
- mourning/grieving
- acceptance and adjustment.

The first two stages have been discussed previously and will not, therefore, be reiterated here, other than to note that there is evidence (albeit somewhat dated) that the denial stage can continue long after the BI survivor has been discharged from hospital (Rape *et al.* 1992). The third stage of emotional turmoil is triggered by the acknowledgement of the permanency of the effects of the injury and the resulting changes to the BI survivor. This turmoil may involve a variety of feelings, including anger, envy, and resentment (of others whose children have not suffered a brain injury), depression, confusion, and guilt (because, for example, of negative feelings towards the BI survivor), bewilderment and anxiety, followed by discouragement and then feelings of being trapped (see Martin 1988). The next stage involves the mourning or working through of the losses the injured child has suffered in terms of (now unobtainable) future goals and roles and changes to his personality. The fifth and final stage sees the acceptance of the deficits of the brain-injured individual and the restructuring of the family by redefining roles and relationships.

Although such models may be of some help in understanding the family response, following BI (Ponsford 1995), they have also been criticized because they are based largely on clinical experience rather than empirical research and are descriptive rather than explanatory (Rape *et al.* 1992). In addition, some families appear to vacillate between stages and may even bypass one or two stages but then get 'stuck' for long periods in another stage for reasons which remain unclear.

There has also been considerable debate concerning the final two stages of mourning and adaptation. Even following a death in the family, mourning may be complicated and may not occur at all, may follow expected patterns, or may be prolonged (Rape *et al.* 1992). For a number of reasons, the mourning process can be further complicated following brain injury. The child may be considerably changed but he is still alive, resulting in the term 'mourning in the presence of the departed' being coined (see Muir *et al.* 1990).

Parents can also feel guilty about mourning the losses their child has suffered and believe they should just be grateful he is alive. In addition, no ceremony is held as there is after a death at which grief can be publicly displayed and shared. Furthermore, the losses suffered by the brain-injured child may not be noticed by others. If they are, expressions of sympathy, which are common following a death in the family, may not be made for fear of upsetting parents. Finally, the survivor of brain injury can show occasional changes which may occur even years after the injury. Thus, uncertainty about recovery can be prolonged. This is particularly likely to be the case for children, given that they will continue to gain skills, acquire knowledge, and develop physically. Williams (in Williams and Kay 1991) suggests that the mourning process in families after a member has had a BI can best be described by the term 'episodic loss reaction'. Reactions are triggered by events such as a memory of the injured child as he used to be or by various milestones. Such milestones may be the anniversary of the injury or a milestone that the person will now never achieve, such as graduate from college. The number of reminders of what was, or could have been, can be considerable and may include old school reports, sporting certificates and trophies, and almost certainly includes photographs. Parents will also often be able to see their child's friends in the neighbourhood reach milestones, such as starting to date, going to college, getting a job, learning to drive, getting married, and having children, that the brain injured child may never achieve. Although it may be possible for parents to predict certain events that are likely to precipitate a loss reaction (such as anniversaries) and make plans accordingly, they may be caught unawares at times, such as seeing one of their child's friends driving a car. Williams (in Williams and Kay 1991) argues that families gradually acquire coping strategies to deal with loss reactions, and that a balance is achieved when the person with the disability is no longer the focal point of the family but all members have their needs met. Different families may, however, use different coping strategies and there may be periodic cycles of adjustment, disequilibrium, and re-establishment of a new balance. It is important to realize that considerable harm can be done if a final 'acceptance' by the family of the survivor's disabilities is demanded by professionals (Kay and Cavello 1994).

Family counselling/therapy

Work with the family may be directed at the feelings of turmoil and loss described previously. It has been suggested (Muir *et al.* 1990) that the distinction between family counselling and therapy is as follows. The aim of supportive family counselling is to provide family members with the opportunity to express feelings of guilt, anger, sadness, and loss and so *possibly* resign themselves to the survivor's disabilities and the potential consequences for themselves. Such help aims to improve day-to-day functioning rather than explore severe or long-term conflict between family members. In contrast, the goals of family therapy are:

- to obtain an in-depth assessment of the family system so that interventions can be tailored accordingly
- to provide a supportive environment in which family members can feel free to express their feelings about the BI and the consequences for themselves
- to educate the family about the nature of their interaction or communication problems and develop methods for resolving conflicts
- to evaluate, clarify, and, if necessary, restructure roles and responsibilities.

There has been some discussion within the literature concerning the need for family therapy following BI. Although it might be thought that most families would only need supportive counselling, the basic structure of the family system in terms of communication, roles, and transactional patterns can be altered when a member suffers a brain injury, and so formal therapy might be indicated. Such fundamental changes may, however, be more likely to occur following BI to an adult in the family than injury to a child. Although it has been suggested that family counselling/therapy can be valuable following brain injury, a note of caution has also been sounded (Brooks 1991). Within family therapy, symptoms are usually seen as reflecting family dysfunction. Following BI, however, such symptoms may be due to the injury rather than other factors, and intervention without examining this possibility may lead to therapeutic failure and result in parents feeling blamed. This is not to say, however, that following such an injury family factors cannot be linked to the child's behavioural problems. For example, temper outbursts may be linked to both the brain injury and the parent's response to the outbursts (see Jacobs, in Williams and Kay 1991).

Family counselling/therapy may be particularly useful in working with the extended family. Grandparents, in particular, often play a considerable role in childrens' lives and are usually extremely upset when their grandson or granddaughter suffers a brain injury. They are often a great source of support and help to parents in the early days following the injury, but may need to take less of an active role as time passes. Negotiation of such role changes can, however, prove difficult. Grandparents may also remain overprotective of the child for longer than parents, causing conflict between them, particularly if the former are still offering respite care to the child.

Cognitive-behavioural interventions

A cognitive-behavioural intervention for parents has recently been described, which proved more effective than a more traditional approach in reducing parental levels of anxiety and depression (see Singer and Powers, in Singer *et al.* [1996] for a full description). The aims of the intervention were to improve coping, provide social support, and reduce psychological distress associated with care-giver stress. Emphasis was on teaching cognitive-behavioural methods for dealing with stress to participants. These included relaxation skills, challenging depressive thoughts, identifying and utilizing social support, and discussion about allowing certain times and places for expressing strong emotion related to grief and loss. Cognitive coping with shattered assumptions, i.e., beliefs about a just world and invulnerability, was also discussed. This type of intervention clearly merits further evaluation.

Refusal to accept psychological help

Families often seem to refuse services which do not appear to be directly geared towards helping the injured child, and it can be difficult to engage the family in formal therapy following the child's discharge from the rehabilitation unit. There may be a number of reasons for this (Foster and Carlson-Green 1993). A central reason, however, may be that the parents need to try to recapture their own sense of control and efficacy without professional assistance, after having lost control during the acute care and rehabilitation stages. As well as regaining 'control' over the child, parents may need to regain control over other aspects of their lives, particularly in terms of work and social links. Thus, the parent who has had to miss a lot of work during the acute and rehabilitation phases may need to concentrate on this aspect. To do so emotions may have to be consciously regulated and even suppressed. Parents may fear that attendance at family sessions would result in them being overwhelmed by feelings and thus make such conscious regulation more difficult. In addition, the injured child may still occupy much of the parents' time and energy, whilst the culture in which the parents exist may be against psychological help. Accepting such help may therefore risk alienating others at a time when their support is badly needed. Thus, it is important that refusal of psychological help by family members is not seen as being necessarily 'pathological' or 'difficult'.

REFERENCES

Beresford, B. A. (1994). Resources and strategies: How parents cope with the care of a disabled child. *Journal of Child Psychology and Psychiatry*, **35**, 171–209.

Bragg, R. M., Klockars, A. J., and Berminger, V. W. (1992). Comparison of families with and without adolescents with traumatic brain injury. *Journal of Head Trauma Rehabilitation*, **7**, 94–108.

Brooks, D. N. (1991). The head-injured family. *Journal of Clinical and Experimental Neuropsychology*, **13**, 155–88.

The impact of brain injury on the family   229

Deaton, A. V. (1986). Denial in the aftermath of traumatic head injury : its manifestations, measurement and treatment: *Rehabilitation Psychology* **31**, 231–40.

Deaton, A. V. (1987). *Pediatric head-trauma: A guide for families.* Healthcare International, Austin, TX.

DePompei, R. and Williams, J. (1994). Working with families after TBI: a family-centred approach. *Topics in Language Disorders*, **15**, 68–81.

Eiser, C. (1993) *Growing up with a chronic disease.* Jessica Kingsley Publishers, London.

Foster, M. A. and Carlson-Green, R. (1993). The transition from hospital to home: family readjustment and response to therapeutic intervention following childhood-acquired brain injury. *Family Systems Medicine*, **11**, 173–80.

Gronwall, D., Wrightson, P., and Waddell, P. (1990). *Head injury: the facts.* Oxford University Press, Oxford.

Kay, T. and Cavello, M. M. (1994). The family system: impact, assessment, and intervention. In *Neuropsychiatry of traumatic brain injury* (ed. J. M. Silver, S. C. Yudofsky, and R. F. Hales) , pp. 532–67. American Psychiatric Press, Washington.

Kreutzer, J. S., Gervasio, A. H., and Camplair, P. S. (1994). Primary care-givers psychological status and family functioning after traumatic brain injury. *Brain Injury*, **8**, 197–210.

Lezak, M. D. (1988). Brain damage is a family affair. *Journal of Clinical and Experimental Neuropsychology*, **10**, 111–23.

Martin, D. A. (1988). Children and adolescents with traumatic brain injury: Impact on the family. *Journal of Learning Disabilities*, **21**, 464–70.

Muir, C. A., Rosenthal, M., and Diehl, L. N. (1990). Methods of family intervention. In *Rehabilitation of the adult and child with traumatic brain injury* (ed. M. Rosenthal, E.Griffith,, M.R. Bond, and J. D. Miller) F.A. Davis, Philadelphia, PA.

Orsillo, S. M., McCaffrey, R. J., and Fisher, J. M. (1993). Siblings of head-injured individuals: a population at risk. *Journal of Head Trauma Rehabilitation*, **8**, 102–15.

Perrot, S. B., Taylor, H. G., and Montes, J. L. (1991). Neuropsychological sequelae, family stress, and environmental adaptation following pediatric head-injury. *Developmental Neuropsychology*, **7**, 69–86.

Ponsford, J. (with Sloan, S. and Snow, P.) (1995). *Traumatic brain injury: rehabilitation for everyday adaptive living.* Laurence Erlbaum Associates Ltd, Hove.

Raines, S. R. and Waaland, P. (1992). *Understanding traumatic brain injury: for kids only.* RRTC Press, Medical College of Virginia, Richmond.

Rape, R. N., Busch, J. P., and Slavin, L. A. (1992). Towards a conceptualization of the family's adaptation to a members head injury: a critique of developmental stage models. *Rehabilitation Psychology*, **37**, 3–22.

Rivara, J. B. (1994). Family functioning following paediatric traumatic injury. *Paediatric Annals*, **23**, 38–43.

Rivara, J. B. , Fay, G., Jaffe, K., Polissar, N., Shurtleff, H., and Martin, K. (1992). Predictors of family functioning one year following traumatic brain injury in children. *Archives of Physical Medicine and Rehabilitation*, **73**, 899–910.

Rogers, P. M. and Kreutzer, J. S. (1984). Family crises following head injury: a network intervention strategy. *Journal of Neurosurgical Nursing*, **16**, 343–6.

Singer, G. H. S., Glang, A., and Williams, J. M. (ed) (1996). *Children with acquired brain injury. Educating and supporting families.* Paul H. Brookes Publishing Co., Baltimore, MA.

Taylor, H. G., Drotar, D., Wade, S., Yeates, K., Stancin, T., and Klien, S. (1995). Recovery from traumatic brain injury in children: the importance of the family. In *Traumatic head injury in children*, (ed. S. H. Broman and M. E. Michel), Oxford University Press, New York.

Waaland, P. and Kreutzer, J. (1988). Family response to childhood traumatic brain injury. *Journal of Head Trauma Rehabilitation*, **3**, 51–63.

Wade, S., Drotar, D., Taylor, H. G., and Stancin, T. (1995). Assessing the effects of traumatic brain injury on family functioning: conceptual and methodolgical issues. *Journal of Pediatric Psychology*, **20**, 737–52

Williams, J. and Kay, T. (ed.) (1991). *Head injury: a family matter*. Paul H. Brookes Publishing Co., Baltimore, MA.

12

Prevention of brain injury

Jackie Gregg and Richard Appleton

The number of patients with serious disability or death from brain injuries is not likely to decrease solely because of better medical care. Prevention is the only cure. This chapter will focus on the prevention of traumatic brain injury i.e. head injuries, but will also discuss the importance of preventative measures in non-traumatic injuries.

PREVENTION OF PRIMARY BRAIN INJURY

Accidents in children and young people are a major cause of death and serious disability and so it is not surprising that reduction in accidents was identified as (and still remains) a major target area in the Health of the Nation (1992) – 'The consequences of some accidents can be life-long disability, or a predisposition to ill-health later in life. Action to reduce accidents will have a significant effect on the health and well-being of children' (Health of the Nation (1992) p. 117).

The Consumer Safety Unit at the Department of Trade and Industry regularly collects data on the essential characteristics of home and leisure accidents from a sample of hospitals throughout the UK. Accidents in the home are more common in children under 5 years of age. Among older children, leisure accidents are more common, with falls and road-traffic accidents being the main causes. In this group there is frequently a clear and direct correlation with both sex (more males injured) and socio-economic deprivation (Platt and Pharoah 1995).

Strategies for accident prevention

Multidisciplinary local child accident prevention committee

The health needs of school-age children (report, Polnay 1995) recommend such a committee should be established in every district to coordinate policy and planning. This will need to involve many agencies, including representatives from the police, road-safety officers, teachers, home safety officers, health education officers, and health personnel. The latter should include community paediatricians, health visitors, school nurses, public health and doctors from accident and emergency (A&E) departments.

Avery and Jackson (1993) list the following as the necessary steps in successfully addressing 'prevention':

- analyse the problem
- determine preventable factors
- specify and plan intervention
- allocate responsibility
- implement a programme
- evaluate effectiveness
- revise the intervention programme.

As an accident involves a child coming into contact with a harmful agent under a defined set of environmental circumstances, prevention involves:

- education
- modifying or removing the agent
- changing the environment.

Effective use of local accident data

School. Data should be fed back to school nurses and school doctors as well as the schools themselves as an essential element in the health profile of the school. Feedback of these data are important in increasing awareness and providing an appropriate local focus for teaching programmes in schools.

To effect environmental changes. Data can be analysed to look at clustering of accidents and steps taken to remove obvious accident 'black spots'.

Targeting 'at risk' groups. Information fed back to health visitors for preschool children and school nurses for school children can be used to discuss accident prevention with individual children and their parents. Those who have suffered an accident are at increased risk and males are more at risk than females (Ohn *et al.* 1995). Health visitors are also important in identifying those children who may be 'at-risk' from non-accidental injury, and in monitoring children who have already been abused and are on the 'at risk' or child-protection register.

Safety education in schools

For Pupils. Pupils in school are a captive audience. Any health promotion and accident prevention education programme carried out as part of the school curriculum is potentially a very useful and effective way to reach all children. A programme of safety education throughout the school years can address age-specific risks at the most appropriate time. Teaching should include risk assessment, managing risk, and risk avoidance. Schools can set examples by ensuring that school playgrounds are safe, by teaching children to swim, providing premises for cycling proficiency instruction, and ensuring that children have assistance to cross roads safely outside school where children are often at their most vulnerable.

Unfortunately, no matter how good the education programme, altering behaviour may be much more difficult. The local strategy groups need to implement programmes which have been proven to be effective. There is still much research to be done in this field.

For Parents. Schools try to involve parents in support of their academic teaching and could involve parents as part of the safety education programme. Parents' groups should be encouraged to promote safety for children in the local community.

School nurses and doctors are a useful resource. In Liverpool, school nurses teach children basic resuscitation techniques and life support.

The Child Accident Prevention Trust

The trust was created in 1979 and is an extremely useful resource and information service for those working in accident prevention. An important part of its work is carrying out research, usually in response to specific accident problems which have been brought to the Trust's attention by government departments, health professionals, and other organizations. (Jackson *et al.* 1988).

Falls

Areas for intervention:

- safety in the home
- safety outdoors
- risky behaviour.

Falls are a common cause of injury in preschool children and usually occur in the home with falls downstairs, out of windows, and out of buggies (Carter and Bannon 1995). Some arise as a consequence of normal development occurring when a child is exploring his environment. It is important that this environment is safe and that serious consequences of normal play are avoided.

Health visitors and community medical staff have a key role in advising parents of specific dangers in the home and of warning parents of potential dangers as each developmental milestone is reached. It is important to give parents a more accurate explanation (and therefore understanding) of the complexity of different tasks and the developmental limitations of children, particularly those under 10 or 11 years of age.

Appropriate use and fitting of approved safety devices such as stair gates and window locks can prevent falls. Baby-walkers need to be used under supervision. Housing young families in high-rise apartment blocks is clearly undesirable for many reasons, including safety.

Particular risks for outdoor play are falls from playground equipment. The energy generated in a fall and transmitted to the brain is related to both the height of the equipment and the energy-absorbing potential of the surface on to which the child falls. The severity of injuries can be decreased by reducing the likelihood of falls (if at all possible), lowering the height of equipment, and by using materials such as sand, wood chips, and rubber under equipment and on the playground surface. Obviously these surfacing materials must be appropriately laid and maintained to be effective.

Young people (particularly boys) frequently indulge in risky and danger-ous behaviour such as climbing trees and onto roofs and falls from these are common. Many boys (particularly in deprived areas) seem to enjoy taking part in games of 'dare' or 'chicken' – trying to cross roads (including dual carriageways) just in front of, or just behind cars, or attempting to jump on to or off already moving vehicles. Schools and parents have a clear role in teaching children about dangerous activities, the risks involved, and their avoidance.

Road traffic accidents

Pedestrians

Areas for prevention:

- children   – road training skills
- parents and adults – setting good examples
                      – age appropriate supervision of children
- drivers   – safe driving
                      – awareness of unpredictability of children
- environment   – traffic-calming measures
                      – pedestrian-only areas
                      – safe play areas
- cars   – safety issues in design.

Pedestrian injuries are a leading cause of childhood mortality and severe brain injury. There has been a fall in mortality for children of all ages, although there are marked international differences. Greatest reductions have occurred in Denmark and Sweden where a greater emphasis has been given to environmental approaches to prevention, compared to New Zealand and Britain where reductions have been less impressive with the focus on prevention having been through education. Legislative changes in Denmark and Sweden have given greater priority to pedestrians. Environmental changes resulted in lower vehicle speeds in urban areas, local streets were designated as 'living areas', and traffic-calming measures such as speed humps were used to encourage compliance. Major roads passing through towns were also modified to reduce traffic speed (Roberts 1993). Conversely, some legislation has actually increased both the risk and incidence of injury to pedestrians. One specific example was the law in North America allowing vehicles to turn right on a red light; child-pedestrian injuries increased by 30% following adoption of this law.

More determined and effective measures to separate pedestrians from traffic could, and should, be undertaken. A significantly higher accident rate occurs in deprived areas, where children of all ages are to be found playing in the streets, often in dangerous or illegal activities and usually unsupervised (Kendrick 1993). Even if there are local parks or safe play-grounds, children will need safe routes to reach them unless supervised or accompanied by adults. Both parks and playgrounds may conceal other risks, including broken bottles, discarded needles, and other dangerous rubbish which may either decrease their use by children, or increase the risk of further injuries, or both.

Safer design of cars could, and should, be addressed. A recent trend for four-wheel drive vehicles to have bull-bars fitted as a fashion accessory has been shown to be associated with increased morbidity and mortality. Car manufacturers should incorporate ABS braking into all their models. Drink driving laws could, and again should, be more strenuously enforced as should the road-worthiness of all motor vehicles. This would require the commitment to divert resources to make this possible.

Pedestrian skills training programmes can improve childrens' behaviour on the roads (Thomson *et al.* 1992). Parents and adults need to be made aware that young children have clear developmental limitations in their ability to safely negotiate traffic. They have an inability to perceive and assess distances and speeds, which combined with natural impulsiveness, results in unsafe traffic behaviour among children younger than 11 years of age (Rivara 1994). Motor immaturity in the younger child may result in delayed reaction times to dangers, further contributing to the risk of injury. Adults need to be educated to show good examples to children.

Car passengers

Areas for prevention:

- safe driving
- seat belts
- car design.

Safe driving to reduce the occurrence of an accident is self-evident. Should an accident occur, then use of seat-belts and suitable child restraints can significantly reduce injury to passengers. There is recent evidence indicating that the incidence of head injuries could be significantly reduced (by almost 40%), if all children travelling in cars used seat restraints or a child safety seat (Ruta *et al.* 1993). Additional data arising from this same study population revealed (perhaps not surprisingly), that a driver with points on the driving licence was over five times more likely to have had an accident resulting in an injury (including a head injury) to a child travelling as a passenger in the car, than a driver without points (Narayan *et al.* 1997).Legislation exists regarding use of front and rear seat-belts (Box 12.1). However, for children to be appropriately restrained in cars at all times, seats have to be available at affordable prices and be easy to use. Many authorities promote the use of car restraints by providing a loan scheme for young children.

BOX 12.1 Legislation regarding use of front and rear seat-belts			
	Front seat	*Rear seat*	*Responsibility*
Child under 3 years	Appropriate child restraint must be worn	Appropriate child restraint must be used, if available	Driver
Child 3–11 years	Appropriate child restraint must be worn, if available, if not, adult seat belt to be worn	Appropriate child restraint must be used, if available, if not, adult seat belt if available	Driver
Child 12–13 years and above	Adult seat belt must be worn, if available.	Adult seat belt must be worn, if available	Driver

Some safety-conscious car manufacturers are introducing child seats specifically designed for their makes of car, which should reduce the risk of the seats being incorrectly fitted/positioned. Devices such as air bags and safety-door locks for children can all help to reduce injury. Rear seat-belts must be fitted in all cars manufactured or sold since 1986.

Cyclists

Areas for prevention:

- children   – wearing of cycle helmets
                                       – cycle skills training

- drivers   – cyclist awareness
                   – safe driving
- environment   – cycle routes
                   – traffic-calming measures
- parents   – adequate supervision
                   – setting good examples
- cycles   – roadworthy, with working brakes and front and
                   rear lights.

Cyclists of all ages are clearly at risk on busy roads. Appropriately manufactured cycle helmets can help reduce injury and it is claimed that they may reduce the risk of head injuries by 85% and the risk of brain injury by 88%; however, to be effective they have to be worn – and worn correctly. Teenage cyclists in Oxford believed in the efficacy of helmets, but only 18% wore one on every cycling ride. Cost was an issue, as was looking ridiculous and being hot and uncomfortable. In addition, the boys believed that their cycling skills would prevent them from injury (Joshi *et al.* 1994).

Role-modelling by mountain-bike athletes, as seen in the televised 1996 Olympic Games, may help to promote cycle helmets as an essential part of cycling equipment. Of course, helmets will not protect against other injuries. Programmes to promote cycling skills and parental supervision for younger children need to be developed and used together with the promotion of traffic-calming measures and an expansion of cycle routes.

Near drowning

Areas for intervention:

- children should be taught to swim
- swimmers should be adequately supervised
- pools and ponds should be fenced off or appropriately covered
- young children should not be left unattended in baths.

The risks of drowning or near drowning vary with the density of water hazards in any child's environment. Children may suffer injury in baths, pools, ponds, rivers, lakes, sea, vehicle immersions with child occupants, from child abuse, and alcohol-related water accidents involving teenagers. Private swimming pools and garden ponds are becoming increasingly popular and pose a great risk particularly to the younger child.

Education must be directed at the need to fence off pools and to have ponds fenced or covered with a grill or grid. Children should be taught to swim from an early age and also given instruction in life-saving skills. Use of appropriate life-jackets and buoyancy aids should be employed for children in boats (of any size and type) with adults being made aware of the dangers. Everyone must be advised on the importance of providing adequate supervision wherever and whenever children are swimming.

Drowning of young children in the bath remains a problem and the dangers of leaving a young child unattended in the bath need to be explained to parents. This is particularly important if the child has epilepsy or any physical disability.

Smoke inhalation

House fires involving children are common, with many children dying and others suffering significant brain injury. Clearly, the danger of fire itself, but also the specific hazards and risks of matches, cigarettes, and flammable materials, as well as the use of fire alarms, need to be promoted – both generally and in schools.

Sports injuries

All sports, contact or otherwise, may cause injury. The risks of serious head injury are greatest in horse-riding, rugby, boxing, and even golf (from a club or ball). Young people need to be made aware of the risks involved and how to enjoy their sports safely. Adequate supervision and training in how to participate safely in these sports is obviously important.

Child abuse

Not all brain injury is accidental and Hobbs (1989) estimated that over 95% of serious intracranial injuries occurring during the first year of life are the result of physical abuse. Non-accidental injury remains a significant cause of head injury beyond the first year of life and throughout childhood. Survivors may be left with a chronic disability (physical, cognitive, emotional, or all three) and epilepsy.

The Area Child Protection Committee (ACPC) provides the focus and forum in each local authority to bring together all those involved with abused children to address child protection. One of the main tasks of the ACPC is to scrutinize the progress on work to prevent child abuse and make recommendations to responsible agencies to identify children at risk and to, hopefully, prevent injury (Area Child Protection Committees 1991).

Infective agents

Areas for prevention:

- ensure high uptake of vaccination against serious diseases (where it exists)
- parental awareness of early signs of serious illness
- medical awareness of early signs of serious illness.

Common childhood infectious illnesses such as measles, whooping cough, and *Haemophilus influenza B* infections can, by causing meningitis or encephalitis, or through metabolic/respiratory complications, result in brain injury. Fortunately, effective vaccines are available to prevent these illnesses. Fear of brain injury from the whooping cough vaccine, which started in the 1970s resulted in low uptake of all vaccines. Much has been done at national and local levels to restore confidence in the vaccination programme, in particular, stressing that the risks of brain damage from the illnesses themselves are far higher than following vaccination or immunization. The primary health care teams have an important role in promoting vaccination and immunizing children and most districts have vaccination and immunisation strategy groups to maintain a high uptake and herd immunity.

Unfortunately, vaccines are not (yet) available for all the serious illnesses of childhood, including meningococcal group B meningitis and septicaemia. Although this particular infection is relatively uncommon, it is important to educate parents and doctors to recognize the early symptoms and signs of infection, so that prompt medical treatment can be initiated and thereby reduce the risk of death and severe brain injury.

PREVENTION OF SECONDARY BRAIN INJURY

As already stated in the opening chapter, a significant amount of ultimate brain injury or damage is caused not by the primary injury itself (whether traumatic or non-traumatic), but by secondary injuries (Chestnut 1995). These secondary injuries are usually caused by a chain reaction or cascade of processes which often produce irreversible damage to brain cells, leading to cell death. The majority of these processes are usually biochemical but may also be immunological. As well as inducing or initiating destructive changes some of these processes may also be involved in attempting to repair damaged cells and tissues. These chain reactions or processes may begin minutes or hours after the initial primary insult or injury and may evolve over hours, days, or even weeks; once initiated these reactions are difficult to terminate. The first hour after the primary head injury (in the case of a traumatic injury) is considered by many to be the crucial time to try and prevent these chain reactions – and secondary damage – from occurring and because of this, it is often called the 'golden hour'.

Numerous attempts and measures have been employed in both this 'golden hour' and in subsequent hours to prevent or at least reduce the incidence and risks of secondary damage. Some of these measures have been shown to be beneficial whilst others are still in the experimental stage and are largely unproven.

General measures

Although the acute management of head (and other brain) injuries has improved recently, it is frequently suboptimal with potentially preventable factors contributing to further brain damage and neurological impairment.
1. Enabling rapid, appropriate, and effective resuscitation by the establishment of paramedic ambulance crews and the delivery of doctors to the site of the accident (whether traumatic or non-traumatic) either by road or by air
2. More appropriate and rapid transfer of brain-injured children following initial stabilization; transporting unstable patients may cause further brain damage (Gentleman and Jennett 1981; Sharples *et al.* 1990).
3. Improved intensive-care facilities to maintain general homeostasis (i.e. to ensure that the following parameters are kept, or are returned, to normal: blood pressure, tissue oxygenation, body temperature, fluid balance, blood glucose levels, etc.) (Chestnut 1995).

Specific measures (usually, but not invariably, targeted at the brain)

1. Hypothermia – nursing the child at a lower body temperature (to 32 or 30°C) to reduce some of the biochemical cascade processes and prevent increases in intracranial pressure (Lyeth *et al.* 1993). Animal studies have shown conflicting results; early studies suggested that hypothermia may exacerbate the release of chemicals (called excitatory neurotransmitters and free radicals) which could predispose to secondary damage, whilst more recent evidence suggests that hypothermia may reduce subsequent neurological damage and dysfunction (Lyeth *et al.* 1993).
2. Anticonvulsants to prevent continuing seizure activity which can cause secondary metabolic damage to the brain and further brain-cell death
3. Pharmacological (drug) treatments – it is known that a number of chemicals may be released from the brain cells as a result of the primary brain insult – whatever the cause (Smith *et al.* 1995). These include:

- excitatory neurotransmitters (principally glutamate, kainate and glycine)
- calcium
- opiate peptides
- catecholamines (adrenaline and noradrenaline)
- free radicals – these are particularly toxic to brain cells and free-radical release is increased by the presence of iron within the cells. The iron itself is released into the cells as a breakdown product of blood, following haemorrhage or bleeding within the brain. Frequently, this bleeding is not in the form of a large blood clot which can be seen on brain-imaging (either CT or MRI) but in the form of multiple small haemorrhages, which are difficult if not impossible to see on brain imaging and which have

resulted from a shearing or tearing effect between cells and small capillary blood vessels within the brain

- nitric oxide
- proteases
- cytokines (including interleukins).

A number of drugs or other chemical compounds have been (and continue to be) developed to try and prevent the release of these chemicals, or at least to reduce their effect and so minimize any secondary brain damage:

- magnesium (sulphate or chloride)
- NMDA (*N-m*ethyl *D-a*spartate) receptor blockers or antagonists, including drugs such as MK801 and ketamine
- vitamins A and C, tocopherols, and other antioxidants – particularly to try and 'mop up' or absorb any free radicals
- calcium channel-blockers or antagonists
- TRH (thyrotropin releasing hormone)
- amphetamines

There are many other approaches (including other chemicals or 'drugs') which are currently undergoing research in animal models of both traumatic and non-traumatic brain injury – most of these are known only by a series of letters and numbers! It must be stressed that these, as well as the specific ones mentioned above, are still largely unproven in preventing or at least reducing secondary brain injury and, importantly, a number may also affect the function of normal, undamaged cells, as well as abnormal, damaged cells. In addition to identifying any therapies which could arrest or even reverse any destructive processes, it would also be important to discover therapies which could enhance reparative ones. It may be many years before any compound or drug is found which is both effective – and 'safe' – and which can be used in the narrow window of opportunity after the primary injury has occurred but before any secondary injury has become irreversibly established.

REFERENCES

Area Child Protection Committee. (1991). In Working Together, Under the Children Act 1989, pp. 5-8. HMSO, London.

Avery, J.G. and Jackson, R.H. (1993). *Children and their Accidents*. Edward Arnold, London.

Carter, Y.H. and Bannon, M.J (1995). Admission due to accidents in preschool children: a local study in North Staffordshire. *Maternal and Child Health*, **20**, 51–6.

Chestnut, R. M. (1995). Secondary brain insults after head injury: clinical perspectives. _New Horizons_, **3**, 366–75.

Gentleman, D. and Jennett, B. (1981). Hazards of inter-hospital transfer of comatose head-injured patients. _Lancet_, **2**, 853–5.

Health of the Nation. (1992). _A strategy for health in England_, pp. 102–15. HMSO. London.

Hobbs, C.J (1989). Head injuries. In _ABC of child abuse_ (ed. R. Meadow), pp. 12–14. BMJ Publications, London.

Jackson, R.H., _et al._ (1988). The work of the Child Accident Prevention Trust. _Archives of Disease in Childhood_, **63**, 318–20.

Joshi, M.S., _et al._ (1994). Cycle helmet wearing in teenagers – do health beliefs influence behaviour? _Archives of Disease in Childhood_, **71**, 536–9.

Kendrick, D. (1993). Prevention of pedestrian accidents. _Archives of Disease in Childhood_, **68**, 669–72.

Lyeth, B. G., Jiang, J. Y., and Liu, S. (1993). Behavioural protection by moderate hypothermia initiated after experimental traumatic brain injury. _Journal of Neurotrauma_, **10**, 57–64.

Narayan, V.K.M., Ruta, D., and Beattie, T. (1997). Seat restraint use, previous driving history, and non-fatal injury: quantifying the risks. _Archives of Disease in Childhood_, **77**, 335–8.

Ohn, T.T., _et al._ (1995). Pattern and risks of accidental injuries in children presenting to a paediatric accident and emergency department. _Maternal and Child Health_, **20**, 404–7.

Platt, M.J and Pharoah, P.O.D. (1995). Child health statistical review. _Archives of Disease in Childhood_, **73**, 541–8.

Polnay, L. (1995). _Health needs of school uge children_. Report of a Joint Working Party. Chairman : L. Polnay. BPA, London.

Rivara, F.P. (1994). Epidemiology and prevention of pediatric traumatic brain injury. _Pediatric Annals_, **23**, 12–7.

Roberts, I.G. (1993). International trends in pedestrian injury mortality. _Archives of Disease in Childhood_, **68**, 190–2.

Ruta, D., Beattie, T., and Narayan, V.K.M. (1993). A prospective study of non-fatal childhood road traffic accidents: what can seat restraint achieve? _Journal of Public Health Medicine_, **15**, 88–92.

Sharples, P. M., Storey, A., Aynsley-Green, A., and Eyre, J. A. (1990). Avoidable factors contributing to death of children with head injury. _British Medical Journal_, **300**, 87–91.

Smith, D. H., Casey, K., and McIntosh, T. K. (1995). Pharmacologic therapy for traumatic brain injury: experimental approaches. _New Horizons_, **3**, 562–72.

Thomson, J.A., Ampofo-Boateng, K., Pitcairn, T., Grieve, R., Lee, D.N., and Demetre, J.D. (1992). Behavioural group training of children to find safe routes to cross the road. _Britsih Journal of Educational Psychology_, **62**, 173–83.

13

A parents' view

This brief chapter gives a detailed (and unedited) account of how one family perceived and coped with their daughter's severe brain injury. The account begins with her arrival on the neuro-rehabilitation ward.

Lizzy was 10 years old when she and her father were involved in a serious collision with another car. Both suffered severe head injuries and a loss of consciousness, although Lizzy's was the more serious, necessitating transfer by helicopter to the neurosurgical intensive-care unit in Walton Hospital. Computerized tomography of her head revealed marked cerebral oedema and a large subdural haematoma which required surgical intervention and evacuation; despite this the cerebral oedema deteriorated and at one point it was felt that she would not survive. Lizzy required ventilatory support for almost one month and after 5 weeks was transferred to the neuro-rehabilitation ward at Alder Hey, under the care of the head-injury rehabilitation team (HIRT).

Twelve months following the accident, Lizzy had made a quite remarkable recovery and was able to recommence full-time education in her local primary school; her secondary school education was (understandably) deferred for 1 year. She had a very mild right hemiparesis, minimally dysphonic speech, an impaired (but rapidly improving), short-term memory, and subtle emotional lability; she had not experienced any early or late post-traumatic epileptic seizures.

The members of the HIRT, in order of appearance in this account by Lizzy's parents, are as follows:

Debbie	– staff nurse and Lizzy's primary nurse on the neuro-rehabilitation ward
Nick	– senior house officer in paediatric neurology
Julie and Helen	– play therapists
Richard	– consultant in paediatric neurology
Gill	– nursing sister
Eileen, Juliet, and Jo	– physiotherapists
Charlie	– Lizzy's dad
Colin	– clinical psychologist
Bronwen	– occupational therapist
James	– Lizzy's older brother

Heather	– physiotherapist responsible for hydrotherapy
Theresa	– staff nurse
Siobhan	– speech and language therapist
Janice	– nutritionist
Sydney	– senior sister, neurosurgical intensive-care unit
Heather	– link teacher between the hospital school and the HIRT
Ian	– physiotherapist.

The team feel that this chapter is as important as all the preceding chapters as it not only reflects a family's view and impression of the rehabilitation process but also demonstrates the parents' role as key team-members in this process.

'We arrived on D3 in early autumn. Lizzy had come by ambulance and we were greeted by our named nurse, Debbie, who had visited us in the Walton Centre before we transferred. After the ordered hush of intensive care, D3 was a bit of a shock. The noise level was unbelievable – televisions blaring, radios playing, children running about. We could barely hear what was being said to us. Lizzy was checked in by Debbie and Nick, a doctor from the rehabilitation team. We listed Lizzy's injuries: some chest congestion, open tracheostomy wound, a suspected fractured pelvis, and a large pressure sore on her heel as a result of a back slab put on in A&E for a broken ankle. These we reeled off as minor problems because for us they were. The real cause of our trouble was underneath the large scar running, like a hairband, across her forehead just above the hairline. Lizzy had required brain surgery to remove a clot, but more importantly, she had suffered severe concussive damage to her brain. Her brain had continued to swell over 48 terrible hours. She nearly died. Luckily she survived, but she had sustained severe brain injury as a result. In the 5 weeks we spent in intensive care we had no response whatsoever from Lizzy, and frankly, we had been told to expect very little in the way of recovery.

Everyone we met in the rehabilitation team seemed very upbeat, cheerful, and positive, which was important because by this time we were totally drained. To meet people that did not seem appalled by Lizzy's condition was a great relief. It made us feel that perhaps Lizzy was not the worse case they had ever seen. Perhaps there was some hope. A phrase coined that day was to become a mantra 'Anything we can get is a bonus'; true – anything is always better than nothing.

The orthopaedic team checked out Lizzy's pelvis and said that it would be safe to move her. This was what the rehabilitation team wanted to hear because what Lizzy needed was movement and stimulation to get through to her and gain a response. We welcomed the news because at last some positive steps were being taken to 'wake Lizzy up'. Or at least that was what we thought we wanted. The play therapists said they would take Lizzy to the Light Room, and so they arrived with a wheelchair and put Lizzy into it. It was at that moment that the reality of our situation hit me. In the quiet, cushioned environment of intensive care, when Lizzy was asleep I could almost pretend that she was alright, that nothing had happened to her; but when she was put into a wheelchair and sat up for the first time since the accident, I could no longer pretend anything. Our beautiful, talented, lively daughter was a blank-faced, floppy stranger who could not even sit normally. Her head lolled and her body could not even bend properly to take the shape of the chair. It was awful. Her blank, open eyes somehow seemed so much worse when she was sitting up. To put someone into a wheelchair who could not even sit properly seemed risky. We drew courage from Julie and Helen. If they thought it was alright – then so be it.

We went off together to the Light Room – a multi-sensory room with soft cushions, moving coloured lights, and music. As we went along the long hospital corridor we tried not to notice the horrified, pitying glances of other parents and patients. Even in hospital there is a scale of awfulness, and we were obviously near the top. Again we felt cushioned by the presence of Julie and Helen whose cheerfulness protected us. Once in the Light Room, Lizzy was put on a large floor cushion and Julie tried to get her to focus on an object and follow it with her eyes. We stared hard at Lizzy, willing her to do it, but she just stared blankly ahead and we felt that she had failed some important test. Briefly, Lizzy seemed to look long and hard into Julie's eyes and then she drifted off again.

In the early stages of Lizzy's treatment we were terrified that they would give up on Lizzy if she did not respond to the various therapies. As we were never sure what they were looking for, this remained a vague fear that we were frightened to articulate in case it precipitated a negative reaction. Quite early on we had 'the talk' with the consultant. We were ushered into the office with Richard and Gill, the ward sister, and we solemnly examined the scans which were every bit as depressing as we expected them to be. We knew that things were bad but it is still difficult to hear it spelled out. The real problem, of course is that nobody knows what kind of recovery you are going to get until you get it. Scraps of information like 'most of what you are going to get comes back in the first 6–12 months' become ridiculously important. The clock is ticking. We had better get cracking. We had heard of rehabilitation being referred to as 'therapy for parents'. The phrase 'Anything we can get is a bonus' hung in the air.

One area of rehabilitation we felt completely comfortable with was physiotherapy. Eileen and Juliet had assessed Lizzy on her first day. Every day after that initial assessment we had a physiotherapy session, and we looked forward to them. Lizzy had been given some splints for her feet to stretch the hamstrings, which had shortened after so long lying down, in preparation for her standing and walking. Just to hear someone considering the possibility of Lizzy standing or walking was cheering. The early exercises were aimed at making Lizzy easier to handle. What made physiotherapy so good for us was that we could watch and pick up any response. Juliet and Jo had Lizzy pushing away a balloon. She appeared to have voluntary movement on her left side. If they asked her to bridge we could see if she was doing as she was asked. Also, we were able to participate in the therapy. We could continue with small exercises like bending her knees and moving her feet up and down for the odd 10 minutes throughout the day, or putting her splints on for an hour, morning and afternoon. Lizzy had to spend an hour or so per day in a standing frame to strengthen her legs and we were shown how to put her into the frame and this became our job. We felt there was something definite we could do to help. Therapy for parents?

By this time we were in a side room because Lizzy had a MRSA (methicillin-resistant *staphylococcus aureus*) infection. The news initially had come as a blow because it meant that she was not allowed out of her room so she was unable to take advantage of all the rehabilitation facilities around the hospital – like the light room, hydrotherapy pool, and the occupational therapy unit. The positive side was that we had a room to ourselves, which meant we had some control over the noise level and our own personal space so we were less inhibited about stroking, cuddling, and talking to Lizzy.

The play therapists also visited daily. They were always bright and cheerful, coming in with 'Right Lizzy, I want you to . . .'. Often their visits would coincide with the time Lizzy was in her standing frame, so a table was fixed onto it during play sessions. Often the sessions appeared impromptu and comprised of bowls of sand, paper, and rice for Lizzy to touch and feel, or objects like keys and toys for her to pick up; we even had musical instruments and tapes for us all to play and sing to. Later, I realized that these 'play sessions' were far more organized than they had appeared to be, but because they were 'play' we were less anxious about Lizzy acquitting herself well. One of the most memorable times for me was when Julie asked Lizzy to lift a plastic football off the table and Lizzy managed it. We felt like cheering. Another time Julie arrived with some paints and asked Lizzy to paint a line on some paper. Initially she did not cooperate, but Julie persisted and eventually Lizzy drew a line and tossed the brush back to Julie as if to say 'There, I've done it – now leave me alone'.

We had been given a chair with Velcro supports around Lizzy's middle and chest to keep her in a reasonably stable sitting position. Often, as she was sitting or standing, she would bang her arms on the chair and roll her head. Her face would pucker up as though she wanted to cry. It seemed that she did not like being moved about or made to do things, but the therapists plugged on regardless. Sometimes we wondered if we should stop them as Lizzy was obviously agitated, but we let the therapists carry on because we believed that they had Lizzy's best interests at heart. They so obviously cared about Lizzy and wanted her to get better we felt we had to follow where they led. Charlie was often braver about this than I was.

We were referred to Colin, a clinical psychologist attached to the team. We found our sessions with him of enormous benefit as we could articulate our fears and ask the questions about head-injury recovery that we wanted to ask. It was too difficult to ask the doctors and therapists who were directly involved with Lizzy the questions we really wanted to ask. Questions like: was her recovery going according to plan? Was Lizzy reaching the milestones that pointed towards a good recovery? Our questions would inevitably be loaded with unspoken pleas for reassurance and that would have been an unfair burden to place upon them. Also, we knew that it was never really possible to predict completely how each patient would respond, so there were no easy answers anyway. With Colin, we could be honest about our wish for reassurance and he gave us general information about the usual patterns of head-injury recovery which, because he was not directly involved with treating Lizzy, we did not load with extra significance.

Lizzy also had occupational therapy in her room and during these sessions we experienced a couple of memorable milestones. Firstly, Bronwen asked Lizzy to build a tower of small bricks. This she did, painstakingly slowly, using her more obedient left hand while I held the brick pile steady. When she had built the tower, Bronwen asked her to knock it down. Lizzy did not respond. Charlie asked her to take the tower down instead, and this she did, taking the bricks off one at a time and placing them in the box. I remember thinking 'That's Lizzy'; Lizzy would think what's the point of building a tower only to knock it down again. The second incident was when Bronwen came in with some pencils and crayons and put a pencil into Lizzie's fist and asked her to make a mark on a piece of paper. Slowly, very slowly, Lizzy manipulated the pencil out of her fist and into her old pen grip between her fingers. I watched, fascinated, thinking 'That's Lizzy – Lizzy is in there somewhere?

Once the MRSA cleared up we were allowed out and about again. Lizzy was taken with other children to the circus. James, her big brother, was to go with her. During this time James had remained at home with his grandparents, so we felt this was an opportunity to include James as he had been rather isolated from us and what had been going on. Lizzy was put into her chair and wheeled off to the minibus. She did not like it. She rolled her head and banged her fist on the chair, her face puckered up, and she was making whiny, gasping noises. We worried about landing James with the responsibility but the nurses took James in hand and had him operating the wheel-chair hoist. We were told firmly that all forms of stimulation were beneficial and off she went. We went to the pub.

Now Lizzy was no longer infectious we could resume the hydrotherapy. Lizzy was put into plastic pants, as she was still doubly incontinent, and a swimming costume. Once in the water, we saw Lizzy automatically move her legs as though she was kicking to swim. Another magic moment. Heather took over the hydro-sessions and they were wonderful to watch. Lizzy had suffered from spastic rigidity and in the warm, soothing water we could almost see her relax and her muscles lose some of their tension.

On November 5th, Helen arranged a little firework party with some of the children from the neurology wards. Again Lizzy became agitated. She did not like going out – after so long indoors, to go out into the fresh air was probably quite frightening. Charlie let off some fireworks in the field at the top of the hospital. Lizzy remained very unhappy and agitated. Later, Lizzy said that this was her first conscious memory.

Now Lizzy was beginning to cooperate more fully and each day brought more improvement. We were getting more facial response and she was managing to smile. I feel I ought to remember her first smile but I don't. As Theresa, one of our nurses, put it; 'The light had come back to her eyes'. She was clearly understanding more of what was going on around her and the pace of her recovery picked up. We had more sessions with the speech therapist, Siobhan, who concentrated on arranging systems of communication for Lizzy as she was still unable to speak. Pictures were given to her so that she could point to them to answer questions. We were able to see that her understanding was good. It appeared that she still had her reading skills so a chart was made with a few words bed, sleep, television, yes, no, mummy and daddy – written on it so that she could point to them to indicate her wishes. Nobody said anything, but when we asked we were told that speech usually returned before reading skills they but were not unduly worried. Lizzy was back with us – we were already in 'bonus'. It was possible that 15 days on a ventilator had probably caused some soreness.

Siobhan was also in charge of whether Lizzy could eat. Up to this point Lizzy had been fed by a nasogastric tube, and in order to establish whether she could eat or drink safely, she had a videofluroscopy. The first videofluroscopy test that Lizzy had undergone had made her agitated and she had not cooperated. It was felt she was unable to swallow liquids safely so Siobhan had said that she could only have solids. That came as a surprise as I had expected Lizzy to start on liquids and work her way up to solids, but liquids are harder to manage in the mouth and are more easily inhaled or aspirated. We had a few videofluroscopies over the weeks and Lizzy's success improved as she became more aware and able to take instructions.

Once Lizzy was allowed solids we had another visit from the nutritionist. Janice had already helped us sort out Lizzy's feeding routine. She had been pump-fed at night to ensure that she got the necessary nutrition and was on a high calorie diet as she had lost a lot of weight. To be fed through the night is unnatural and attempts were made to introduce bolus feeding during the day. As these took time to administer, they often interfered with therapy times which we considered to be more important. So the pump-feeding continued longer than was usual. Once Lizzy could eat she was asked to express her food preferences. As she pointed to various pictures of food, we rather sheepishly admitted to a rather poor, child-led diet. It was the effort that was made to give Lizzy food that she could enjoy eating that highlighted the general wish to coordinate all Lizzy's therapies and give her positive and encouraging experiences. Even appealing food could be a positive force for recovery. If she liked what she was eating she would try to feed herself. As we spoon-fed Lizzy I was reminded of what Sydney, the sister in intensive care, had said: 'It is as if you have been given a newborn. Everything must be learnt again. I haven't got a crystal ball. I can't tell you how much she'll be able to learn'. As we progressed through feeding, toilet-training, and learning to walk and talk again, I realized what she had meant.

By December, Lizzy was well enough and ready to be sent to the hospital school. She was lukewarm about going as she was still in a wheelchair and could not speak. To be among other children and in a schoolroom environment was, however, another step towards normality. Heather, the school's link teacher, introduced Lizzy and us to the school and its staff. Once at school, she was treated with the same caring, good humour that she had experienced everywhere else and she became reconciled to going. Her first spoken word - 'home' – was uttered when we were given the news that we were to be allowed home for the night. I was a bit scared driving her home as she seemed so vulnerable. I couldn't bear the thought of anything happening to her after all she had been through.

Soon we were allowed home for good. We were to come back three times a week for various therapy sessions. As we continued to go about the hospital, things were very different from our earlier experiences of the hospital corridor. We were greeted by the many people we had come into contact with and everyone took real pleasure in seeing Lizzy getting better and better. We continued to attend physiotherapy for sessions of sitting, standing, balancing and walking with Juliet and Ian. We went to Bronwen for sessions to improve Lizzy's poor short term memory and manual dexterity and also to Siobhan to get Lizzy's voice louder and to improve her vocal range. Eventually, our normal life at home began to take up more of our time and our sessions were cut to 1 day a week. As Lizzy returned to her old school it became obvious that we could not continue to make the journey to Liverpool, and arrangements were made to return to our own area and community services. We said goodbye to the team with real regret and immeasurable gratitude.

We still attend the occasional out-patient appointment. On one visit I heard a nurse remark as Lizzy walked in 'That's not bad for someone who was never going to do anything'. I felt for the first time that perhaps it wasn't such a bad thing that in the early days we were not burdened with too much information and a specific prognosis based on early clinical evidence. The team had done the right thing. On the basis of 'Anything we can get is a bonus', they had quietly got on with the job and gone for everything they could get.

Further reading – general

Avery, J.G. and Jackson, R.H. (1993). Children and their accidents. Edwards Arnold (division of Hodder and Stoughton), London.

Becker, D. P. and Gudeman, S. K. (ed.) (1989). Paediatric head injuries – special considerations. In *Textbook of head injury*. WB Saunders, Philadelphia.

Broman, S. H. and Michel, M. E. (1995). *Traumatic head injury in children*. Oxford University Press, New York.

Johnson, D. A., Uttley, D., and Wyke, M. (1989). *Childen's head injury: who cares*? Taylor and Francis, London.

McLaurin, R. L. and Rouban, R. (1990). Diagnosis and treatment of head injury in children. In *Neurological surgery* (ed. J. R. Youmans), pp. 2149–93. W B Saunders, Philadelphia.

Rivara, F. P. and Barber, M. (1985). Demographic analysis of childhood pedestrian injuries. *Pediatrics*, **76**, 375–81.

Ylvisaker, M. (1985). *Head-injury rehabilitation: children and adolescents*. Taylor and Francis, London.

Appendix: Useful organizations

CHILDREN'S HEAD INJURY
TRUST (CHIT)
c/o Neurosciences Unit
The Radcliffe Infirmary
Woodstock Road
OXFORD
OX2 6HE
Telephone/fax: 01865 224786

HEADWAY
The National Head Injuries
Association
7 King Edward Court
King Edward Street
Nottingham
NG1 1EW
Telephone/fax: 0115 924 0800

THE FAMILY FUND
Beverley House
Shipton Road
York
YO1 2ZX
Telephone: 01904 21115

BRITISH EPILEPSY ASSOCIATION
Anstey House
40 Hanover Square
Leeds
LS3 1BE
Telephone: 0113 243 9393
Fax: 0113 242 8804
Helpline (free): 0800 309030

MERSEY REGIONAL EPILEPSY
ASSOCIATION
Glaxo Neurological Centre
Norton Street
Liverpool
L3 8LR
Telephone: 0151 298 2666

EPILEPSY ASSOCIATION OF
SCOTLAND
48 Govan Road
Glasgow
G51 1JL
Telephone: 0141 427 4911

NATIONAL SOCIETY FOR
EPILEPSY
Chalfont Centre for Epilepsy
Chalfont St Peter
Buckinghamshire
SL9 0RJ
Telephone: 01494 873991

Index